Endoscopic
Neurological Surgery

Endoscopic Neurological Surgery

Editor

David F Jimenez MD FACS
Professor
Department of Neurosurgery
University of Texas Health Science Center
San Antonio, Texas, USA

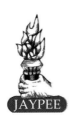

The Health Sciences Publisher

New Delhi | London | Panama

Jaypee Brothers Medical Publishers (P) Ltd

Headquarters

Jaypee Brothers Medical Publishers (P) Ltd
4838/24, Ansari Road, Daryaganj
New Delhi 110 002, India
Phone: +91-11-43574357
Fax: +91-11-43574314
Email: jaypee@jaypeebrothers.com

Overseas Offices

J.P. Medical Ltd
83 Victoria Street, London
SW1H 0HW (UK)
Phone: +44 20 3170 8910
Fax: +44 (0)20 3008 6180
Email: info@jpmedpub.com

Jaypee Brothers Medical Publishers (P) Ltd
17/1-B Babar Road, Block-B, Shaymali
Mohammadpur, Dhaka-1207
Bangladesh
Mobile: +08801912003485
Email: jaypeedhaka@gmail.com

Jaypee-Highlights Medical Publishers Inc
City of Knowledge, Bld. 235, 2nd Floor, Clayton
Panama City, Panama
Phone: +1 507-301-0496
Fax: +1 507-301-0499
Email: cservice@jphmedical.com

Jaypee Brothers Medical Publishers (P) Ltd
Bhotahity, Kathmandu, Nepal
Phone +977-9741283608
Email: kathmandu@jaypeebrothers.com

Website: www.jaypeebrothers.com
Website: www.jaypeedigital.com

Endoscopic Neurological Surgery

First Edition: **2019**

ISBN: 978-93-5270-122-3

Printed at: Ajanta Offset & Packagings Ltd., Faridabad, Haryana.

Dedication

This book is dedicated to all the patients
whom I treated with endoscopic
neurosurgical techniques and contributed
to the expanding volume of knowledge
of this surgical discipline

Contributors

David F Jimenez MD FACS
Professor
Department of Neurosurgery
University of Texas Health Science Center
San Antonio, Texas, USA

David N Garza BA MA
Research Coordinator
Department of Neurosurgery
University of Texas Health Science Center
San Antonio, Texas, USA

Michael J McGinity MD
Neurosurgeon
San Antonio
Texas, USA

Colin T Son MD
Neurosurgeon, Meriter UnityPoint
Health and University of Wisconsin
Hospitals
Madison, Wisconsin, USA

Kevin R Carr MD
Neurosurgeon
San Antonio
Texas, USA

Preface

I became very interested and fascinated by the concept of minimally invasive brain surgery during my pediatric neurosurgery fellowship. Very little had been written on the subject, so I approached several of the world leaders in the area and sought their opinions and advice. As my academic career matured over the last quarter of a century, my experience and confidence grew, thereby allowing me to care for many patients and many different clinical conditions. With experience came knowledge and facility of execution. Many "surgical pearls" were learned, developed and adapted over the years. The impetus for writing this book came from the desire to share many of these "pearls" with those interested in the field and who are beginning to embark in its execution. Additionally, it has also been written for those in the medical profession who may be interested in the subject. These include residents, medical students, physician assistants, and nurses. The chapters cover a wide spectrum of clinical problems that are amenable to endoscopic treatment. A review of the literature presents the reader with an overview in each chapter. The actual surgical technique is then described in a concise, simple but yet detailed fashion. I find that carefully executed endoscopic neurosurgical techniques provide the patients with significantly less trauma, morbidity and complications. It is my hope that these techniques are taken up by many more developing surgeons and that many more patients are helped in the process.

David F Jimenez

Acknowledgments

I especially appreciate the constant support and encouragement of Shri Jitendar P Vij (Group Chairman) and Mr Ankit Vij (Group President) of Jaypee Brothers Medical Publishers (P) Ltd, New Delhi, India in helping to publish this textbook and also their associates particularly Ms Chetna Malhotra Vohra (Associate Director—Content Strategy) and Ms Nikita Chauhan (Development Editor) who have been prompt, efficient and most helpful.

Contents

CHAPTER 1

History of Neuroendoscopy

David N Garza, David F Jimenez

INTRODUCTION

Knowing historical facts relating to a specific area, provides the reader with a better understanding and appreciation for the efforts undertaken by previous pioneers. In this introductory chapter, we wish to provide the reader with a glimpse to the past of Neuroendoscopy and how the discipline evolved. Key technical advances made by a few and courageous clinicians/surgeons and their disciples have led to our current state of affairs where we can provide our patients with minimally invasive, safe and successful surgical options.

ENDOSCOPIC PREHISTORY

Endoscopy has existed, albeit in a crude form, since the time of the ancient Egyptians around 1550 BC.[1] Their practice of transnasal excerebration involved the use of hook-shaped rods that helped them peer inside the human nasal cavity and extract cerebral components during mummification. This technique has been postulated by some to be the earliest example of minimally invasive neurosurgery.[2] The approach used by the ancient Egyptians (as depicted by Herodotus in his book *Histories*) is surprisingly similar to modern-day transphenoidal surgery.[1]

The next phase of endoscopic evolution deals with the development of speculum technology. The Talmud, which dates back to 1300 BC, contains a description of a speculum precursor that was used to examine Jewish women in order to determine their eligibility to participate in sexual intercourse.[2] Specula were also used by physicians like Hippocrates between 460 BC and 370 BC.[3] Excavations conducted in Dion, a village located in northern Greece, uncovered bronze instruments that bear a resemblance to the specula used by modern physicians. The instruments from Dion date back to approximately 200 BC; tools of similar construction from around 70 AD have also been recovered from the ruins of Pompei (Fig. 1).

Speculum implementation was advanced by Albukasim of Cordoba (936–1013 AD), an Arabian physician who used reflected ambient light during his examinations to aid visibility.[3] In 1585, Giulio Cesare Aranzi improved on this technique by using closed tubes and mirrors to reflect ambient light into the nasal cavity.[3] This eventually paved the way for the "Godfather" of modern endoscopy, Philipp Bozzini (1773–1809), whose

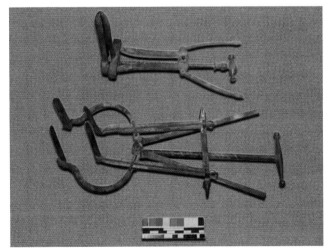

Fig. 1: Ancient Greek specula recovered from the ruins of Pompei, dated around 70 AD.
Source: Reprinted with permission from Elsevier. Abd-El-Barr MM, Cohen AR. The origin and evolution of neuroendoscopy. Childs Nerv Syst. 2013;29:727-37.

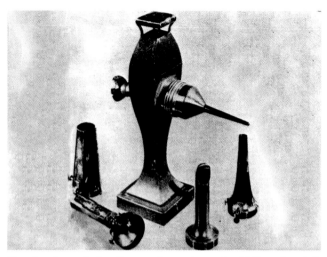

Fig. 2: One of the first endoscopic tools: Philipp Bozzini's "Lichtleiter" or light guide, 1805.
Source: Reprinted with permission from Elsevier. Edmonson JM. History of the instruments for gastrointestinal endoscopy. Gastrointest Endosc. 1991;37:S27-56.

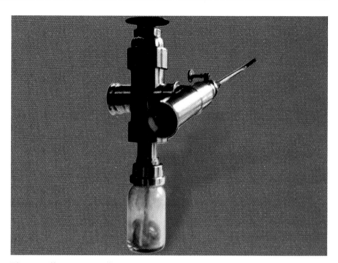

Fig. 3: Illustration depicting Antonin Desormeaux's endoscope. The kerosene lamp at bottom of device burned alcohol and turpentine to fuel illumination.

"Lichtleiter" or "light guide" used a candle as an external light source along with a set of reflective mirrors on one end of the device and various examining tubes that could be fitted to the opposite end.[2]

THE FIRST ENDOSCOPES

Bozzini was hopeful that his endoscopic device (Fig. 2) could be used to visualize body cavities, but he encountered some resistance in the process of trying to legitimize his invention. Although many ecclesiastical prohibitions banning the exploration of human anatomy had been lifted since the Renaissance, the church's influence was still not totally withdrawn from the activities of the scientific community. Church officials halted the progress of Bozzini's invention during its second round of testing when they withheld their approval for the Lichtleiter to be used on live patients.[2] Because of petty rivalries already in place, the device was ridiculed by the Alert Faculty of the University of Vienna and subsequently rejected.[2] Bozzini's work was not appreciated in its time, but his three part design principle of a light source, reflective mirrors, and an investigative eye piece remains a staple guide for the construction of endoscopic technology even within our modern age.

Despite the widespread opposition against Bozzini's invention, there were two individuals who followed his model and tried to improve his work: Pierre Salomon

Segalas and John D Fisher. Their endoscopic instruments resembled the Lichtleiter through the incorporation of a light source, a reflective surface, and a graduated series of tubular specula.[4] Fisher added a double convex lens to sharpen and enlarge the image produced by his endoscope while Segalas modified his scope to visualize bladder stones and then crush them with a lithotrite.[4] Segalas is also noteworthy because his guidance informed the work of the individual responsible for the next major innovative leap in endoscopic design: French urologist Antonin Desormeaux.[4]

Desormeaux is credited with several "firsts" in endoscopic history. In 1853, he designed a scope with a kerosene lamp that burned alcohol and turpentine (Figs. 3 and 4) coupled with a 45° mirror that could reflect that lamp's light into different parts of the body.[3,5] Some scholars consider this cystoscope (an endoscope used specifically for visualizing the urinary bladder through the urethra) to be the first proper endoscope.[6] Desormeaux used this instrument to remove a papilloma from a patient's urethra, which was recognized as the first recorded therapeutic use of an endoscope.[6] He is also credited as being the first person to use the term "l'endoscopie" (endoscopy).[3]

The problem with Desormeaux's device was that while it produced better illumination, the heat emitted from the lamp's galvanized platinum wires was so intense that it could easily burn a patient. German dental surgeon Julius

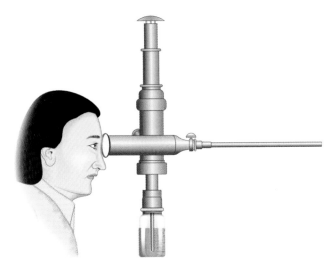

Fig. 4: Illustration depicting the operation of Desormeaux's endoscope.

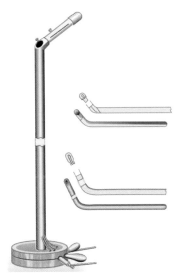

Fig. 5: A prototype of the Nitze-Leiter cystoscope, 1877. *Source*: Reprinted with permission from Elsevier. Herr HW. Max Nitze, the cystoscope and urology. J Urol. 2006;176:1313-6.

Bruck was able to alleviate this problem, in part, when he designed a glass cooling system that diminished heat emission with a stream of water surrounding the platinum filament.[3] It is unclear whether or not Bruck was able to implement his design in a clinical setting, but his cooling system as well as the placement of his light source were both significant contributions to the field.[2] The notion to place a light source inside the human body was particularly important because all sources of light used for endoscopic visualization up to that point in time had been external.

NITZE AND THE MODERN ENDOSCOPE

German physician Maximilian Nitze also recognized the limitations created by external light sources. He wanted to incorporate Bruck's ingenious lighting system into a prospective design, but felt that the endoscope's small field of view still posed a problem for the operator. He supposedly got the inspiration for a solution to this problem while cleaning the eyepiece of his microscope. When he looked out through the lens, Nitze realized that he could see through it clear across to a neighboring church; this observation led him to incorporate a telescoping system into his design in order to obtain a wider field of view.[2] Nitze's concept was a major step in endoscope evolution because it finally afforded the device magnification, a quality all previous systems lacked up to that point

because they were simply tubes that directed light down to their distal tips.[7]

In 1879, Nitze collaborated with Austrian engineer Josef Leiter to produce a cystoscope that used Bruck's water-cooled platinum filament lamp at its distal end along with a series of telescoping optical lenses set inside a metal tube that would relay an image down the scope.[2,3] Although it was the first endoscope to combine all these crucial elements (Fig. 5), the device was still burdened by insufficient illumination, cumbersome usage, and expensive operation costs.[6] Eight years after Thomas Edison's incandescent light bulb became commercially available, Nitze incorporated it into the distal end of his cystoscope, which made the instrument much more manageable and gained the physician widespread acclaim in the process.[2]

NEUROENDOSCOPY EMERGES

Before the 19th century, there were several obstacles in place that hindered the successful application of endoscopy to the field of neurosurgery. For example, compared to the gastrointestinal tract the brain is a much darker organ; it cannot be illuminated sufficiently by ambient sources of light.[8] Another difficulty was that early anatomists had a flawed understanding of neurophysiology that perpetuated misconceptions about cerebrospinal fluid (CSF) and the structure of the brain's cavities.[8] But by the 20th century, substantial work had been done that mapped out the ventricular and subarachnoid spaces and, thanks to Nitze's contributions, physicians were finally equipped with the tools they needed to explore those dark corridors.

Endoscopes were finally used for neurosurgical purposes in 1910, when American urologist Victor L'Espinasse introduced a cystoscope into the lateral ventricle and bilaterally fulgurated the choroid plexus of two infants suffering from hydrocephalus.[9] One patient died postoperatively and the second lived for 5 years before passing.[10] L'Espinasse himself did not seem to think much of the endeavor. He presented his work at a local meeting, but never formally published it.[2] He later wrote the operation off as a sort of novelty, describing the procedure to his daughter, Victoire (also a physician), as "an intern's stunt".[10] Still, in spite of this modest assessment, the long-term impact made by his experimental foray into neurosurgery should not be understated. Readers should not gloss over the fact that the first person to perform neuroendoscopic surgery was not a neurosurgeon, but a young urologist with an unprecedented idea. His example can serve us as a reminder about the importance of innovation and inter-discipline dialogue.

THE DANDY YEARS

Although L'Espinasse deserves credit for being the first person to perform neuroendoscopic surgery, the acknowledged father of modern neuroendoscopy is Walter E Dandy, who used the endoscope in his study and treatment of hydrocephalus. Dandy determined that communicating hydrocephalus could be alleviated by extirpating the choroid plexus. Doing so would reduce the production of CSF, which was out of balance due to an obstruction in the subarachnoid space.[11] In 1918, he published a manuscript describing this extirpation.[11] It was a somewhat crude procedure that required a nasal dilator to keep the cortex open and necessitated that he drain the patient's entire volume of CSF before removing the choroid plexus.[2] The operation left three out of four patients dead within 1 month of treatment; the fourth survived and showed no signs of hydrocephalus 10 months after surgery.[2]

In 1922, Dandy tried to incorporate a cystoscope into these choroid plexectomies.[12] Unfortunately, he was unable to complete the operations without assistance from his nasal dilator and forceps.[8] Though these initial

attempts were not successful, Dandy was steadfast in his efforts. During the same year, he published the first endoscopic observations of the ventricles and coined the term "ventriculoscopy".[9] Dandy was enthusiastic about refining his approach, but admitted that the images created by his ventriculoscope did not surpass in quality those produced by the more routine pneumoventricolography technique.[9] He reluctantly concluded that neuroendoscopy had little to offer brain surgery that could not be achieved through conventional means.[8]

Elsewhere, while Dandy struggled to find a space for neuroendoscopy, progress was being made by his contemporaries. In 1923, William Mixter published the first report describing an endoscopic third ventriculostomy in a patient with noncommunicating hydrocephalus.[13] During the same year, Fay and Grant reported the first black and white photos taken of a child's dilated ventricles, which they took using a cystoscope affixed with a camera.[9,13] In 1936, John Scarff performed an endoscopic plexectomy using a new version of the ventriculoscope made of a tube with an inner stylet connected to irrigation channels that maintained constant intraventricular pressure; this prevented the ventricular collapse that might have contributed to Dandy's poor initial results.[9]

In spite of his skepticism, Dandy did not completely abandon the prospect of endoscopy playing a larger role in neurosurgery. He turned to Howard Kelly (the renowned father of cystoscopy) for design advice and personally directed engineers from the Wappler Electric Co. in order to construct a better ventriculoscope.[8] He also took notice of the advancements made by his peers. In 1934, Tracey J Putnam adapted a urethroscope for endoscopic electrocautery and introduced endoscopic choroid plexus coagulation, a procedure that could successfully obliterate the choroid plexus without the need for resection.[8] The operation was different from Dandy's because the CSF was not completely evacuated from both ventricles before cauterization of the choroid plexus took place.[14] Dandy eventually adopted this coagulation technique when performing his own endoscopic choroid plexectomies; he also used a probe similar to Putnam's that could be threaded through the scope.[8]

By 1945, despite the progress he had made, Dandy ultimately considered the endoscope's neurosurgical application to be restricted to young children with ventricular tumors or older patients with tumors that had accidentally disclosed during choroid plexectomies.[8]

Because he was a prominent surgeon who played such a huge role in pioneering the technique, Dandy's criticism of neuroendoscopy might have contributed to the 20-year period of stagnation that followed.[8] The lack of endorsement was not the only factor, of course. Ventricular CSF shunt surgery and microsurgery both minimized the need for neuroendoscopy to be further explored in the coming generation.

THE DECLINE AND REBIRTH OF NEUROENDOSCOPY

In 1951, Nulsen and Spitz described a treatment for hydrocephalus using ventricular shunt placement.[6] Because it was easier to perform and had lower associated mortality rates than other available techniques, shunting quickly became popular.[12] In the 1960s, the emergence of microneurosurgery also played a role in neuroendoscopy's decline because the microscope provided surgeons with everything the endoscope seemed to lack: high magnification, adequate illumination, and the ability to work in deep structures with little damage to the surrounding tissue.[2] While interest in neuroendoscopy waned during this era, there were several technological advancements taking place that helped set the stage for the field's resurgence in the 1970s. These included the development of fiber optics, the rod-lens system, SELFOC (self-focusing) lenses, and charged-coupling devices (CCDs). Many of these advancements can actually be connected to a single individual: British optical physicist Harold Hopkins. It is primarily because of his contributions that the endoscope became a viable surgical tool after so many years of dormancy.

FIBER OPTICS

In 1951, Hopkins was at a dinner party seated next to a gastroenterologist who complained about the shortcomings of endoscopic technology.[2] Most scopes available at the time followed Nitze's design, which used a series of lenses housed in an air-filled tube. This system engendered several problems for the operator, including color distortion, poor illumination, excessive heat, cumbersome size, and rigidity.[7] While working with research student Narinder Kapany, Hopkins utilized coherent bundles of glass fibers to create the fiberscope, a flexible device with a shaft that could be bent and still conduct an image from one end to the other.[3,7] The glass fibers also permitted the transmission of light without excessive heat.[12]

Although Hopkins was the person who successfully manifested them into a practical tool, some of the concepts that made up his fiber optic technology had already been described by previous researchers. For example, Heinrich Lamm demonstrated that light could be conducted through a bundle of glass fibers in 1932.[7] Daniel Colladon and Jacques Babinet demonstrated the earliest light conductors in the 1840s.[13]

ROD-LENS SYSTEM

Although the advancements produced by Hopkins' fiberscope were helpful, the device was still lacking, particularly when it came to image quality and light transmittance. In 1959, Hopkins was approached by James G Gow, a urologist who wanted to take photographs of the inside of the bladder in order to develop cancer therapies.[3] He needed the current cystoscope improved so that it could provide superior illumination. This prompted Hopkins to develop the rod-lens system, which replaced the large gaps of air in between a series of small lenses that were found in Nitze's endoscope with large glass rods in between a series of small air spaces.[3] This new design allowed those spaces of air to act as a series of thin lenses, which resulted in an all-around superior experience for the user.

The conduction of light in an endoscope is a function of the refractory index of the conducting medium.[7] In the case of Nitze's telescoping design, that medium was air. Hopkins realized that glass has a refractory index that is 1.5 times greater than air. By exchanging glass for air and air for glass, the system's refractory index increased, which significantly expanded the scope's field of vision and light gathering capacity.[7] This adjustment also reduced the diameter of the endoscope, which made it less invasive for patients.[3] The rod-lens system was a crucial innovation in design that made the endoscope so much more effective. It still forms the basis of the rigid endoscopes that are currently used today.[2]

SELFOC LENS

In 1966, Hopkins collaborated with German optical instrument manufacturer Karl Storz to design a rigid endoscope that used a new type of lens: the self-focusing optical (SELFOC) lens.[3] While conventional lenses have a uniform refractive index, the SELFOC lenses contain a gradient index glass with a variable refractive index that changes according to the radial dimension of the lens.[12]

Conventional endoscopes used during this time period required the meticulous placement of relay and field lenses to construct an image. The SELFOC lens technology essentially eliminated the need for relay lenses while creating a wider field of vision and preserving light conduction.[12] Surgeons were able to operate without making large incisions and could peer into body cavities with more clarity than ever before. This refined endoscope was made commercially available in 1967 and marked the technological beginning of modern neuroendoscopy as we know it today.[3]

CHARGED-COUPLING DEVICES

Charged-coupling devices are solid-state devices that are capable of converting optical data and light signals into electrical impulses and digital data.[3,12] They were invented by Willard Boyle and George Smith in 1969 in order to address the question of how to incorporate video camera technology into endoscopic operations.[3] CCDs decreased the size of endoscopic systems and improved the quality of their transmitted images by conducting them over to high-resolution screens.[3]

NEUROENDOSCOPY: YESTERDAY, TODAY, AND TOMORROW

In the 1970s, after decades of disinterest, neurosurgeons started to reconsider endoscopy's role as a surgical tool. This resurgence can be attributed to several factors. Other specialties had already demonstrated the benefits of minimally invasive surgery (shorter convalescence period, lower morbidity rates, and greater patient satisfaction).[15] Endoscopic tools had become smaller and more efficient. They were easier to use and provided superior imaging than their predecessors. Perhaps the main reason why neurosurgeons revisited endoscopy was because of the complications related to CSF shunting, such as shunt malfunction, infection, migraines, and overdrainage.[12] Shunt failure was (and still is) an especially dangerous risk for patients in developing countries because those individuals might live far away from facilities that could repair a faulty shunt.[2] Endoscopic third ventriculostomy is often preferable to shunt surgery because it offers a more physiological solution to the problem posed by hydrocephalus: it allows the ventricular CSF to drain directly into the subarachnoid space.[12]

In 1973, Takanori Fukushima introduced the first flexible neuroendoscope (the "ventriculofibroscope"), which was used to explore treatments related to intraventricular tumor biopsy, cyst fenestration, and hydrocephalus.[9,15] However, it was not until 1994 that Jones and colleagues described an endoscopic third ventriculostomy procedure that had a 61% success rate in treating hydrocephalus.[12] Since that time, endoscopic third ventriculostomy and choroid plexus cauterization have both become popular treatment options for hydrocephalus. Their success recovered neuroendoscopy's once-damaged reputation and suggested to curious neurosurgeons the possibility that this approach could be applied to other areas of surgical interest as well.

Neuroendoscopy is currently being used to treat many other kinds of disorders, including skull base tumors, intraventricular tumors, intracranial cysts, degenerative spine disease, and craniosynostosis.[12] However, some of these applications offer unique obstacles that must be addressed before the field can progress any further. Some of the challenges associated with intraventricular surgery include operating within a fluid medium, achieving hemostasis, performing bimanual microdissection, and maintaining optimized visualization.[13] The development of direct endoscopic visualization (endoscope-controlled microsurgery) will likely facilitate bimanual microdissection and assist in the maintenance of hemostasis for intraventricular lesions.[13] Improvements made to endoscopic instrument design, such as the development of a miniaturized endoscopic ultrasonic aspirator, should also enable surgeons to resect lesions with more accuracy and safety.[13]

Skull base endoscopy is a much younger field than intraventricular endoscopy. While intraventricular investigation rebooted in the 1970s and 1980s, a routine endoscopic approach to skull base pathology was not firmly established until almost 20 years later.[13] Challenges endemic to endoscopic skull base surgery have included demarcating surgical boundaries that are limited by critical neurovascular structures, maintaining hemostasis, losing binocular vision, and developing sufficient skull base reconstruction techniques.[13] Much work has been done to address these limitations so that safe access along a wide arc of the midline skull base from the frontal sinuses to the odontoid process is now attainable.[13]

One of the main reasons why endoscopy is so appealing is because it is minimally invasive. This attribute has been particularly beneficial to peripheral nerve applications, such as carpal tunnel decompressions.[13] Carpal tunnel decompression took off in the late 1980s and is now the operation of choice for many surgeons because of its excellent success rates and low complication rates.[13] Endoscopic approaches have been considered for other peripheral nerve surgeries as well, including ulnar nerve decompressions.[13]

In the future, flexible endoscopes and wireless camera technology could reduce our dependence on the rigid rod-lens system.[13] Robotic endoscopic devices might provide more sophisticated panoramic and circumferential views of the ventricular system and three-dimensional endoscopic technology could potentially compensate for the loss of binocular vision currently associated with contemporary endoscopic technology.[13] Robot-assisted systems might equip surgeons with the ability to perform techniques that could not otherwise be executed in confined spaces like the ventricular system or the paranasal sinus, but one major limitation of such surgery would be the loss of haptic feedback that normally exists during standard procedures.[13] That problem could potentially be overcome, but only with sufficient advancement in haptic sensor and pressure generator technology.

Endoscopic investigation began centuries ago, with vague conceptions and primitive instruments. The field persisted thanks to the tenacity and ingenuity of innovators from various specialties, but its progress was still slow. A practical, reliable endoscope did not emerge until only recently, within the last 60 years. The incorporation of endoscopic technique into routine neurosurgery took time to establish because the first operations that used it were fraught with so much danger and technical difficulty.

After its associated technology improved, neuroendoscopy finally started to build up its reputation. It is no longer merely a feasible technique; in many cases it is the preferred treatment option. Some consider its comprehension to be an absolute necessity for neurosurgeons and suggest that it will soon become the standard of care by which many of today's procedures are performed.[16] Although neuroendoscopy has flourished since the time of its humble origins, with the right technological advancements bolstering it there is still much room left for it to grow, both in terms of general efficacy and surgical application.

REFERENCES

1. Fanous AA, Couldwell WT. Transnasal excerebration surgery in ancient Egypt. J Neurosurg. 2012;116(4):743-8.
2. Abd-El-Barr MM, Cohen AR. The origin and evolution of neuroendoscopy. Child's Nerv Syst. 2013;29(5):727-37.
3. Di Ieva A, Tam M, Tschabitscher M, et al. A Journey into the technical evolution of neuroendoscopy. World Neurosurg. 2014;82(6):e777-89.
4. Edmonson JM. History of the instruments for gastrointestinal endoscopy. Gastrointest Endosc. 1991;37(2 Suppl): S27-56.
5. Lau WY, Leow CK, Li AK. History of endoscopic and laparoscopic surgery. World J Surg. 1997;21(4):444-53.
6. Schmitt PJ, Jane JA, Jr. A lesson in history: the evolution of endoscopic third ventriculostomy. Neurosurg Focus. 2012;33(2):E11.
7. Abbott R. History of neuroendoscopy. Neurosurg Clin North Am. 2004;15(1):1-7.
8. Hsu W, Li KW, Bookland M, et al. Keyhole to the brain: Walter Dandy and neuroendoscopy. J Neurosurg Pediat. 2009;3(5):439-42.
9. Decq P, Schroeder HW, Fritsch M, et al. A history of ventricular neuroendoscopy. World Neurosurg. 2013;79(2 Suppl):S14.e1-6.
10. Grant JA. Victor Darwin Lespinasse: a biographical sketch. Neurosurgery. 1996;39(6):1232-3.
11. Dandy WE. Extirpation of the choroid plexus of the lateral ventricles in communicating hydrocephalus. Ann Surg. 1918;68(6):569-79.
12. Li KW, Nelson C, Suk I, et al. Neuroendoscopy: past, present, and future. Neurosurg Focus. 2005;19(6):E1.
13. Zada G, Liu C, Apuzzo ML. Through the looking glass: optical physics, issues, and the evolution of neuroendoscopy. World Neurosurg. 2013;79(2 Suppl):S3-13.
14. Azab WA, Shohoud SA, Alsheikh TM, et al. John Edwin Scarff (1898-1978) and endoscopic choroid plexus coagulation: a historical vignette. Surg Neurol Int. 2014;5:90.
15. Shiau JSC, King WA. Neuroendoscopes and instruments. In: Jimenez DF (Ed). Intracranial Endoscopic Neurosurgery. Neurosurgical Topics. Park Ridge, IL: The American Association of Neurological Surgeons; 1998. pp. 13-27.
16. Nobles AA. The physics of neuroendoscopic systems and the instrumentation. In: Jimenez DF (Ed). Intracranial Endoscopic Neurosurgery. Neurosurgical Topics. Park Ridge, IL: The American Association of Neurological Surgeons; 1998. pp. 1-12.

CHAPTER 2

Endoscopic Ventricular Anatomy

David F Jimenez

INTRODUCTION

Intimate anatomical knowledge and understanding of the brain's ventricular system is essential and fundamental in successfully treating patients with ventricular pathology. Furthermore, a thorough knowledge of surgical anatomy is a must in order to safely and successfully perform endoscopic ventricular procedures. This chapter aims to familiarize the reader with both anatomical and surgical anatomy of the human ventricles. A detailed description, along with high definition intraoperative endoscopic photographs are presented.

VENTRICULAR SYSTEM

The ventricular system is comprised of two symmetrical C-shaped cavities joined in the middle (Fig. 1A) by the foramina of Monro. The cavities form part of each cerebral lobe: frontal, occipital, temporal and parietal (Fig. 1B). These paired lobal cavities join in the middle to form two single midline ventricles: the third and fourth (Figs. 1A and 1C) which are connected by the aqueduct of Sylvius.[1]

FRONTAL HORN

In order to gain better and more realistic understanding of ventricular anatomy, we will proceed with an imaginary journey. Let's assume that you have been miniaturized to a size of about 10 mm and are able to freely move inside the ventricles. If you stand in the right frontal horn at the level of foramen of Monro and look anteriorly, what do you see? (Figs. 2A and B). The anterior wall of the frontal horn. Straight ahead is the genu of the corpus callosum (CC). Superiorly on the roof is the body of the CC and inferiorly, making the floor, is the rostrum of the CC. Therefore, the CC forms the roof, anterior wall, and floor of the frontal horn. Now look laterally and you will see a gray matter structure bulging into the ventricle. This is the head of the caudate, which makes the lateral wall of the lateral ventricle (Figs. 3 and 4). Looking at your feet, you will see that you are standing on the anterior thalamic tubercle. Looking medially, the foramen of Monro is seen with the columns of the fornix forming its anterior and superior boundaries (Fig. 5). The septum pellucidum is seen extending above the fornix and reaching the undersurface of the body of the CC. On the lower left quadrant of the foramen of Monro, the septal vein is seen coursing superior-inferiorly and the thalamostriate vein coursing lateromedially. The choroid plexus, extending from the ventricular body is seen entering the foramen on its way to the roof of the third ventricle (Fig. 6). Turning around and looking posteriorly one sees that the roof of the ventricle is made up of the body of the CC and the floor by the thalamus. The medial wall is made of the posterior remnants of the corpus callosum. The lateral wall is comprised of the body of the caudate nucleus (Fig. 7).

ANTERIOR THIRD VENTRICLE

If we now walk through the foramen of Monro into the third ventricle and face forward, the anterior portion will be seen (Fig. 8). While standing on the midbrain, looking down and ahead, the mammillary bodies will be seen with the tuber cinereum in front of it (Fig. 9). Further anteriorly a hyper pigmented reddish area of depression will be seen. This is the infundibular recess and the area of

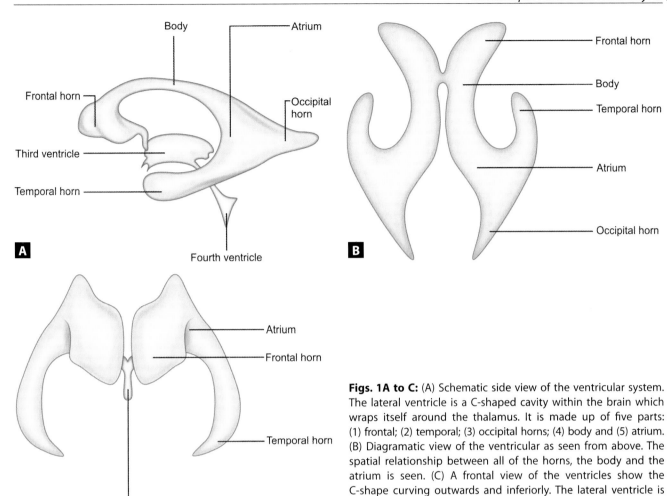

Figs. 1A to C: (A) Schematic side view of the ventricular system. The lateral ventricle is a C-shaped cavity within the brain which wraps itself around the thalamus. It is made up of five parts: (1) frontal; (2) temporal; (3) occipital horns; (4) body and (5) atrium. (B) Diagramatic view of the ventricular as seen from above. The spatial relationship between all of the horns, the body and the atrium is seen. (C) A frontal view of the ventricles show the C-shape curving outwards and inferiorly. The lateral ventricle is connected to the third ventricle via the foramen of Monro.

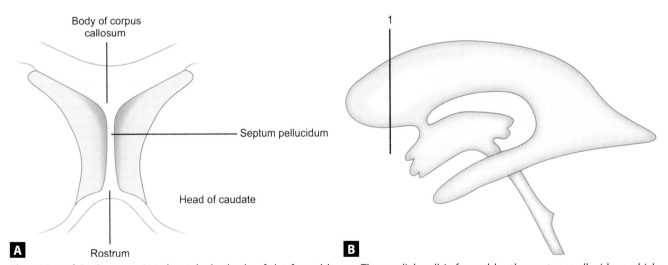

Figs. 2A and B: Cross-section through the body of the frontal horns. The medial wall is formed by the septum pellucidum which extends from the body to the rostrum of the corpus callosum. The lateral walls are formed by the head of the caudate nucleus. The roof by the body and the floor by the rostrum of the corpus callosum. The anterior wall is made up entirely by the genu. [1 refers to the location of the cross-section of Fig. 2A (to the left of Fig. 2B)].

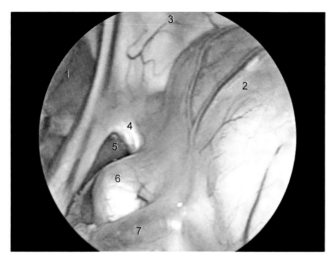

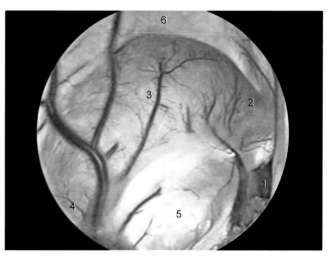

Fig. 3: Patient with longstanding hydrocephalus. The septum pellucidum is absent; (1) caudate nucleus head on left side; (2) caudate nucleus head on right side; (3) genu of corpus callosum; (4) fornix; (5) foramen of Monro; (6) anterior thalamic tubercle; and (7) thalamostriate vein.

Fig. 4: Endoscopic view of left lateral ventricle. (1) Foramen of Monro; (2) head of caudate in the frontal horn; (3) body of caudate; (4) beginning of the tail of the caudate; (5) thalamus; and (6) corpus callosum.

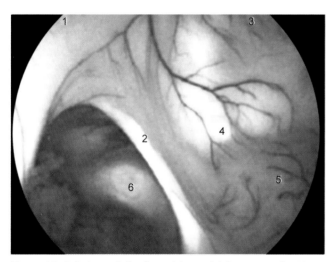

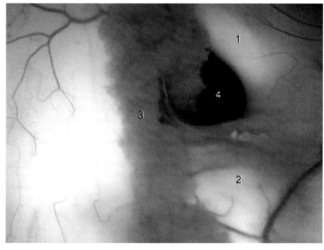

Fig. 5: Medial view of the frontal horn. (1) Septum pellucidum; (2) fornix; (3) genu of corpus callosum; (4) rostrum of corpus callosum; (5) head of the caudate; and (6) posterior aspect of optic chiasm in the anterior third ventricle.

Fig. 6: View of right frontal horn. (1) Fornix; (2) thalamus; (3) choroid plexus; (4) foramen of Monro.

the hypothalamus that produces oxytocin and vasopressin. Looking straight ahead one sees the anterior wall of the ventricle: lamina terminalis. Inferiorly a bulging area of white matter is seen at the inferior most part of the lamina terminalis, the optic chiasm with the suprachiasmatic recess at its junction with the lamina. Superiorly, one sees another band of white matter coursing transversely from fornix to fornix, the anterior commissure.

Laterally the walls of the ventricle are made up by the medial hypothalamus.

POSTERIOR THIRD VENTRICLE

Standing at the level of the foramen of Monro and looking back, the contents of the posterior third ventricle are clearly visualized. The floor is made up by the top

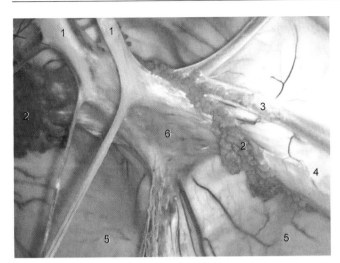

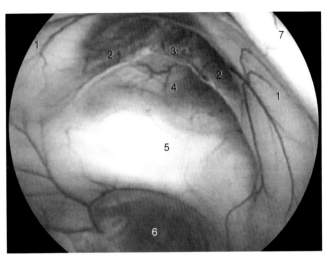

Fig. 7: View of the posterior lateral ventricular system. Both sides are visualized due to chronic absence of the septum pellucidum. (1) Fornices; (2) choroid plexus; (3) thalamostriate vein on right side; (4) thalamus; (5) occipital horns; and (6) superior layer of tela choroidea.

Fig. 8: Endoscopic view through right foramen of Monro. The anterior third ventricle is seen. (1) Medial hypothalamus; (2) anterior cerebral arteries (A1 segment); (3) anterior communicating artery; (4) lamina terminalis; (5) optic chiasm; (6) infindibular recess with its characteristic reddish color; (7) anterior commissure.

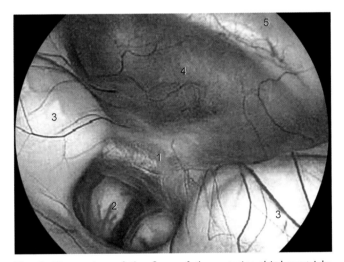

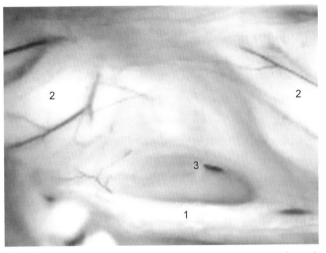

Fig. 9: Direct view of the floor of the anterior third ventricle. (1) The top of the basilar artery; (2) pons; (3) mammillary bodies; (4) tuber cinereum; and (5) posterior clinoid process is seen through the thin tuber cinereum.

Fig. 10: Posterior third ventricle as seen when entering through foramen of Monro. The image is upside down from typical anatomical text views. (1) Posterior commissure; (2) floor made up of mesencephalon (cerebral peduncles); and (3) aqueduct of sylvius.

of the mesencephalon (midbrain) (Fig. 10). The lateral walls are made up by the medial borders of the thalami. Although not always, the massa intermedia, connecting both thalami, will be seen in the middle of the ventricle. The massa is located in the upper half of the ventricle and is present in about 75% of brains (Fig. 11). It is typically located about 4 mm posterior to the foramen of Monro. The roof of the ventricle is made up of four layers: (from inferior to superior) tela choroidea; vascular layer containing the medial posterior choroidal arteries and internal cerebral veins; a neural layer comprised of the body of the fornix and the crura and hippocampal commissure; superior layer of tela choroidea. The velum interpositum is the space between the two layers of tela choroidea in the roof of the third ventricle. It is a closed space that extends

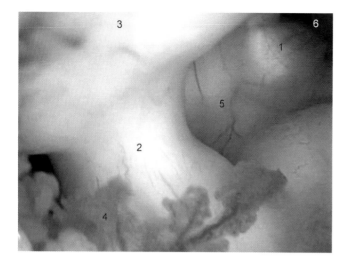

Fig. 11: Third ventricle. (1) Right mammillary body; (2) massa intermedia; (3) left thalamus; (4) choroid plexus; (5) mesencephalon; and (6) tuber cinereum.

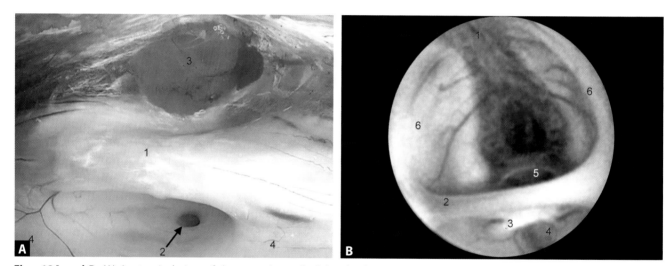

Figs. 12A and B: (A) Anatomical view of the posterior wall of the third ventricle. (1) Posterior commissure; (2) aqueduct of sylvius; (3) pineal gland along with the pineal recess; (4) mesencephalon. (B) Endoscopic view of the roof and posterior wall of the third ventricle as seen from the right foramen of Monro. (1) Choroid plexus under the lower layer of the tela choroidea, making the roof of the third ventricle; (2) massa intermedia between the thalami; (3) posterior commissure; (4) membrane covering the aqueduct of sylvius; (5) pineal gland; and (6) thalami.

from a tapered end at the foramen of Monro to the splenium and posterior wall of the ventricle. The choroid plexus in the third ventricle hangs from the undersurface of the lowermost tela choroidea layer, on the roof of the ventricle. The roof of the third ventricle extends from the foramen of Monro anteriorly to the suprapineal recess posteriorly. The posterior wall of the third ventricle extends from the suprapineal recess superiorly to the aqueduct of the sylvius inferiorly. Following the structures from superior to inferior one sees the suprapineal recess,

the habenular commissure, the pineal gland and its recess, the posterior commissure and the aqueduct of Sylvius (Figs. 12A and B).

BODY OF LATERAL VENTRICLE

By definition the body of the lateral ventricle begins at the posterior edge of the foramen of Monro and extends to the point where the corpus callosum and fornix come together and the septum pellucidum tapers to an end.[2] Looking up one sees that the roof is made up by the

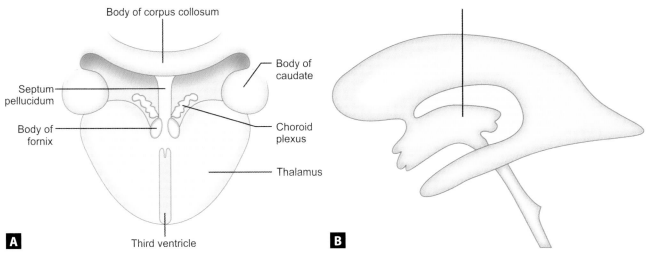

Figs. 13A and B: (A) Cross-section through the body of the lateral ventricle. The roof is formed by the body of the corpus callosum. The floor by the dorsal aspect of the thalamus. The lateral wall by the body of the caudate. The medial wall is made up of the septum pellucidum and the fornix inferiorly. (B) Shows the location of the cross-section in Figure 13A.

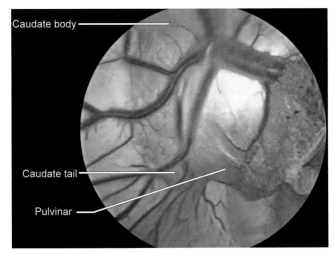

Fig. 14: Left trigone area is visualized. The caudate wraps itself around the thalamus with the body and tail in the atrium.

transversely coursing fibers of the corpus callosum. The lateral walls are formed by the body of the curving caudate nucleus. The medial wall is formed by the body of the fornix. Finally, the floor is made by the dorsal aspect of the thalamus (Figs. 13A and B).

OCCIPITAL HORN AND TRIGONE

The posterior edge of the body of the lateral ventricle is contiguous with the atrium/trigone area (Fig. 14). The roof of the atrium is formed by the corpus callosum and

its component parts: body, splenium, and tapetum. The lateral wall is formed by the tail of the caudate nucleus anteriorly and the tapetum posteriorly.[3] The floor is formed by the collateral trigone, an area that bulges into the ventricle and overlies the collateral sulcus (Figs. 15A and B). The medial wall is made up of two prominences. Superiorly the bulb of the corpus callosum and inferiorly by the calcar avis. The occipital horn extends from the atrium to the tip of the occipital lobe.[4] Similar to the atrium, its medial wall is formed by the bulb of the corpus callosum and the calcar avis (Fig. 16). The floor is formed by the collateral trigone and the roof and lateral wall by the tapetum of the corpus callosum. Although in normal persons the occipital horn is collapsed and invisible, it can expand significantly with ventricular pathology.

TEMPORAL HORN

Like the occipital horn, the temporal horn is normally collapsed and nonvisible but can expand with hydrocephalus and other pathologic conditions. Its margins extend from the atrium of the lateral ventricle to the tip of the temporal lobe behind the amygdaloid nucleus. The roof of the temporal horn is formed by the tapetal fibers of the corpus callosum and the curving tail of the caudate nucleus (Figs. 17A and B). The floor is formed lateral by the collateral eminence and medially by the hippocampal formation. The medial wall is formed superiorly by the inferior surface of the thalamus and tail of the

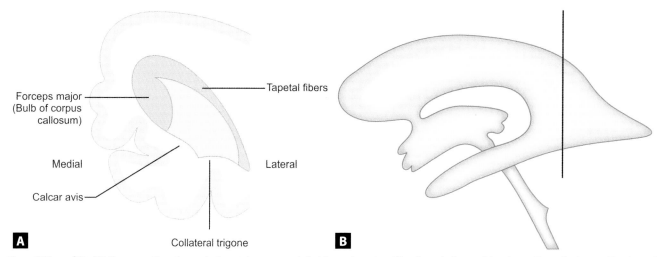

Figs. 15A and B: (A) Cross-section through the atrium an occipital horn junction. The floor is formed by the collateral trigone. The lateral wall and roof are formed by the tapetum. The superior part of the medial wall is formed by the bulb of the corpus callosum which overlies the forceps major and inferiorly by the calcar avis, a prominence that overlies the calcarine sulcus. (B) Shows the location of the cross-section in Figure 15A.

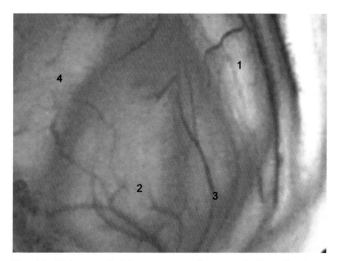

Fig. 16: Right occipital horn as seen from the ipsilateral atrium. (1) Calcar avis; (2) occipital pole; (3) bulb of the corpus callosum; (4) tapetum.

caudate. The inferior medial wall is formed by the fimbria of the fornix. Lastly, the lateral wall is made by the down sloping fibers of the tapetum, which separate the temporal horn from the posteriorly running optic radiations.

FOURTH VENTRICLE

The fourth ventricle is a diamond- and tent-shaped structure located in the posterior fossa between the pons/medulla and the cerebellar hemispheres. It communicates anterosuperiorly with the third ventricle via the aqueduct of Sylvius and posteriorly with the cisterna magna via the foramen of Magendie. The roof has the shape of a tent and is formed by the fastigium at its apex and the superior medullary velum (from fastigium to aqueduct of Sylvius) and inferior medullary velum (from fastigium to foramen of Magendie). The floor of the fourth ventricle is diamond shape and spans the pons superiorly and the medulla inferiorly. It may be divided into three compartments: (1) a superior or pontine part; (2) an intermediate or junctional part; and (3) inferior or medullary part. The intermediate part extends into the lateral recesses and connect with the foramina of Luska. At its most inferior aspect the obex is seen and is closely related to the area postrema. Several prominences are seen on the floor and these include the hypoglossal trigone, facial colliculi, and vagal trigone (Fig. 18). At the midlevel of the floor, thin whitish strands of fibers are seen traveling medial to laterally and are known as the stria medullares (Fig. 19). The choroid plexus is located on the roof of the fourth ventricle.

CONCLUSION

The anatomy of the ventricular anatomy has been described in sufficient detail to assist the surgeon in recognizing the structures during surgery and to help with proper preoperative planning. For those unfamiliar with the anatomy it is recommended that it should be carefully reviewed and studied in anatomical cadaveric specimens.

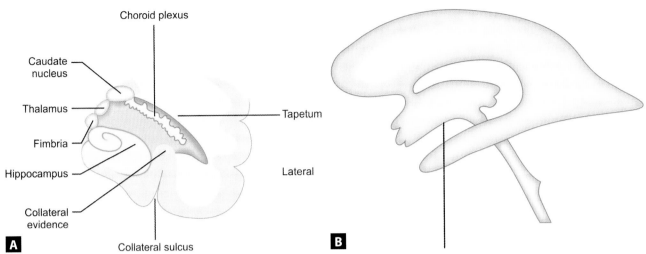

Figs. 17A and B: (A) Cross-section through the temporal horn shows that the floor is divided into a medial portion (prominence overlying the hippocampus) and lateral portion (collateral eminence). The roof is made by the caudate nucleus and tapetum. The medial wall by the thalamus and fimbria. The lateral wall is formed by the tapetum. (B) Shows the location of the cross-section in Figure 17A.

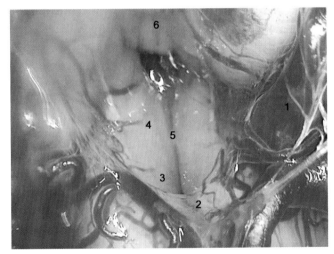

Fig. 18: Lower half of the fourth ventricle. (1) Posterior inferior cerebellar artery; (2) obex; (3) hypoglossal trigone; (4) vagal trigone; (5) median sulcus; and (6) choroid plexus.

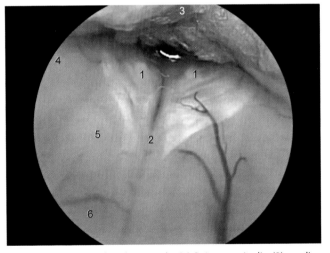

Fig. 19: Floor of the fourth ventricle. (1) Striae terminalis; (2) median sulcus; (3) choroid plexus; (4) vestibular area; (5) vagal trigone; and (6) hypoglossal trigone.

Knowledge of the anatomy is critical for a successful outcome in endoscopic ventricular surgery.

REFERENCES

1. Gardner E, Gray D, O'Rhilly R. Anatomy, A Regional Study of Human Structure, 3rd edition. WB Saunders Co. 53: 603, 1969.

2. Carpenter M, Core Text of Neurosurgery, 2nd edition. Waverly Press; 1978.

3. Wen HT, Rhoton Al. Mussia Surgical Anatomy of the Brain 2:38-62; Youmans Neurological Surgery; 6th edition; Elsevier, 2011.

4. McMinn R, Hutdings R. Color Atlas of Human Anatomy. Yearbook Medical Publishers; 1977.

CHAPTER 3

Endoscopes and Instrumentation

David F Jimenez

INTRODUCTION

The unique nature of the human central system, in terms of anatomical arrangement and complex relationships, requires delicate and individual approaches. Such structural arrangement presents limitations not encountered in other body cavities. To access the ventricular system or other deep cerebral structures requires specialized instrumentation. Although not fully versatile, currently available instrumentation has undergone important recent modifications. Presented in this chapter is an overview of presently available endoscopes and instrumentation used for neuroendoscopic surgery.

OPTICS

Major advancements in optics and scope design have taken since Maximilian Nitze introduced the first lens endoscope in 1877. Nowadays, the rod lens systems of rigid endoscopes, coupled with high definition cameras and monitors, provide the surgeon with superb visualization of the ventricular system. Endoscopic systems are primarily of two types: (1) The rod lens system provides higher resolution imaging with the larger endoscopes providing better images and (2) the other systems are the flexible, fiberoptic scopes, which provide greater maneuverability and flexibility in handling to the sacrifice in resolution. Due to the physical arrangement of the fibers, a significant amount of light is lost, leading to poorer resolution. Additionally, although the fibers can bend, they can also break leading to further image degradation and loss of pixels.

ENDOSCOPES

Endoscopes are produced in many sizes and configurations. Some are made of glass and others from fiberoptic silica glass fibers. Rigid scopes are constructed with solid glass and are therefore nonflexible, non-steerable and non-bendable. Flexible scopes, on the other hand, are steerable, flexible, and maneuverable. The question always arises as to which one is better. Selection of the appropriate endoscope is dependent on procedure type and need. One is not necessarily better than another, depending on the situation and surgeon's preference.

Rigid Endoscopes

The construction of rigid endoscopes may be done in two primary ways: A rod of solid glass or a group of small rod glass units separated with air between the lenses. The latter became the method of choice for mass manufacturing of rigid endoscopes in the 1940s and 1950s. In 1959 Professor Harold H Hopkins, of the University of Reading, designed and patented an elegant solution to the poor resolution of the existing scopes. He reduced the amount of air space between the small rod lenses by exchanging the air for more glass, thus making the lenses longer and mirroring the effect of the air spaces (Figs. 1A and B). Hopkins endoscopes produced higher resolution and greater depth of focus by cutting the tip of the endoscope, the angle of view could be changed from 0° to 30°, 70°, and even 120°. Additionally, by increasing the amount of glass within the endoscopes, Hopkins achieved a significant increase in light transmission due to the higher refractive index of glass versus air. (Refractive index of

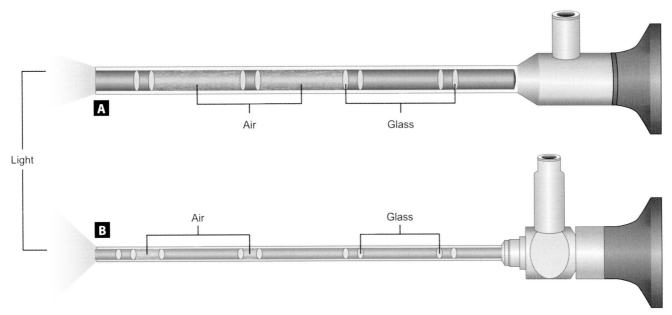

Figs. 1A and B: Schematic diagrams of a typical rigid rod lens endoscope. (A) The original Nitze's endoscope with small rod glass lenses interspaced with larger areas of air spaces. (B) Hopkins' modification of enlarging the glass rods and decreasing the air spaces in between. This led to smaller scopes producing greater illumination.

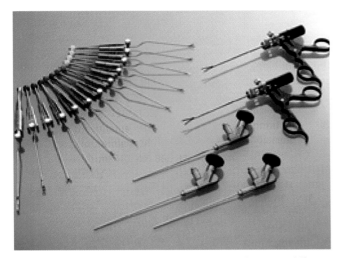

Fig. 2: The rigid endoscope GAAB system showing different angled endoscopes and instrumentation used with the system to perform neuroendoscopic procedures.
Source: Courtesy of Karl Storz Co.

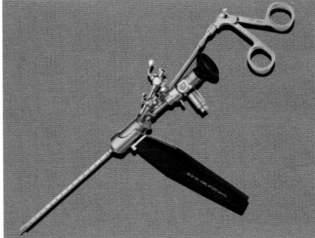

Fig. 3: The Oi HandyPro Endoscope. This versatile scope has a smaller working diameter and is easier to manipulate into smaller compartments or through a narrow foramen of Monro. It has three working parts.
Source: Courtesy of Karl Storz Co.

1.5 vs 1.0). Transmission of light is 50% better through glass than through air.

Karl Storz began producing endoscopes for otolaryngologists in Germany in 1945 and has since then expanded to many other surgical fields. Currently, there are a number of endoscope manufacturers who produce a large

array of endoscopic systems. Storz (Karl Storz, GmbH and Co, KG, Tuttlingen, Germany) perhaps produces the largest variety of endoscopic systems. These include the DECQ, GAAB (Fig. 2), Schroeder, Genitori, Oi HandyPro (Fig. 3), LOTTA (Fig. 4), Frazee, Galzio, Mortini, systems

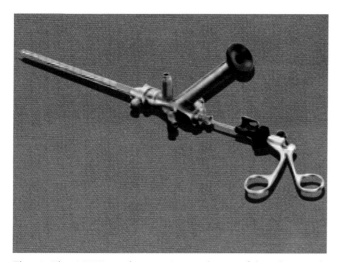

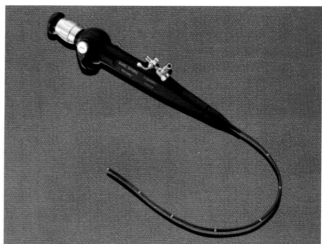

Fig. 4: The LOTTA endoscope is another useful and versatile system which has excellent optics and multiple working channels. *Source*: Courtesy of Karl Storz Co.

Fig. 5: Storz flexible endoscope has 360° freedom of movement when properly manipulated with both hands. It only has a single working port/channel. *Source*: Courtesy of Karl Storz Co.

among others. Other manufacturers include Olympus, Codman, and Medtronic among others.

Flexible Endoscopes

These endoscopic systems are constructed of flexible silica glass and a distal objective lens packaged with multiple light fibers. As such, these endoscopes are flexible and bendable. The image fibers are arranged in a coherent bendable which allows the image to be properly reconstructed on the proximal end of the fiber. The flexible endoscope transmits light across the flexible silica glass fibers. These fibers are coated with a cladding material that has low refractive index. As the light passes from a material of higher refractive index (silica glass) to one of lower refractive index (cladding material), the light encounters optical interference, and as such, degrades by approximately 30%. This of course leads to lower illumination and resolution as a compromise for flexibility. The larger the flexible scope, the better the illumination and resolution (as in those used by pulmonologists and gastroenterologists). However, due to the size and highly delicate architecture of the brain, neurosurgeons utilize smaller endoscopes, which produced degraded images. As with rigid scopes, several companies produce these scopes. The typical neuroendoscope has a diameter between 2.8 mm and 4 mm and carries a single working channel and working lengths of 34–40 cm and total lengths between 64 cm and 70 cm. Working channel

diameter vary between 1.2 mm and 1.5 mm. The tip of these endoscopes can be flexed anywhere between 120° and 170° (Fig. 5).

Disposable Endoscope

In the late 1990s, technology advanced to the point where small, fiberoptic disposable endoscopes were first introduced by the Claris Corporation. Currently Medtronic (Minneapolis, MN) produces a group of disposable endoscopes that provide the neurosurgeon with improved access and flexibility. The NeuroPEN endoscope is ideal for placing ventricular catheters in the desired location and under direct visualization. The outer diameter (OD) is 1.14 mm and the endoscope fits inside the ventricular catheter. The tip of the ventricular catheter can be cut to provide a slit opening (there are catheters available with manufactured slit tips) (Figs. 6A and B) through which the endoscope can be advanced and the catheter can be placed in the desired location (Fig. 7). Additionally, this endoscope has an irrigation port which provides for clearing of any debris and improves visualization. Another flexible and disposable endoscope is the Murphy Scope (Fig. 8) of slightly larger OD (2.3 mm) the endoscope has a flexible metal housing which can be manipulated and bent in any desired shape to reach tight spaces. I have used this scope inside the spinal cord when treated multi-loculated or septated syringomyelia with great success. It also has an irrigating port which allows for

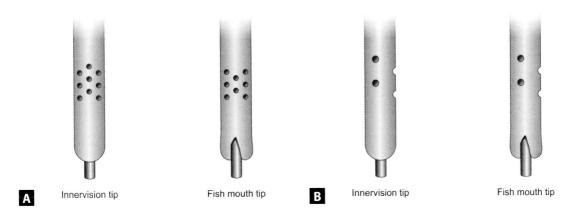

| A | Innervision tip | Fish mouth tip | B | Innervision tip | Fish mouth tip |

Figs. 6A and B: Tip of a ventricular catheter with a NeuroPEN endoscope inside of it. The scope can be advanced in front of the tip via two different types of catheters: (1) Innervision or (2) fish mouth. The catheter can then be placed in the desired location under direct visualization.

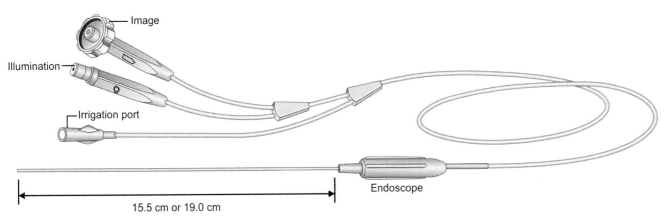

Fig. 7: NeuroPEN neuroendoscope illustration showing the entire system. This disposable scope has a coupler for a camera and light source as well as a single irrigation port. Irrigation is very useful particularly when placing the ventricular catheter in small ventricles or cysts.

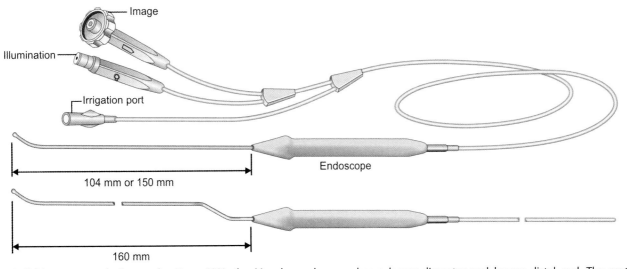

Fig. 8: With a set up similar to the NeuroPEN, the Murphy endoscope has a larger diameter and longer distal end. The metal surrounding the optical fibers is malleable and as such the tip may be bent in any direction or angle.

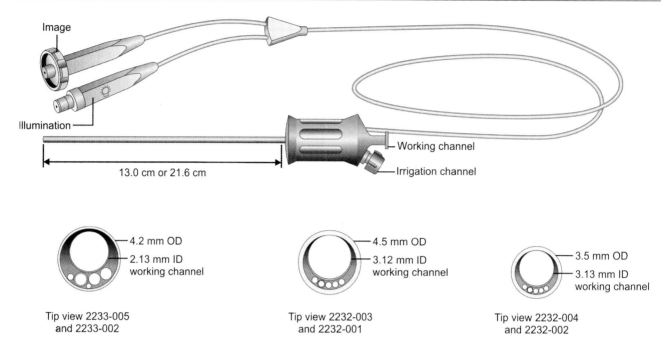

Fig. 9: The channel scope is manufactured with different outer diameters (3.5 mm, 4.2 mm, and 4.5 mm). Likewise, the working channel comes in varying diameters and has an irrigating proximal port as well.

better visualization and hydro dissection of tissue (Fig. 8). Lastly, a larger more rigid endoscope (the Channel endoscope, Medtronic) with an outer diameters ranging between 3.5 mm and 4.5 mm are also available. These scopes have working channels with internal diameters ranging between 2.13 mm and 3.12 mm. Also equipped with irrigating channel, these endoscopes provide adequate access and visualization (Fig. 9). Although the resolution is significantly less than that of rigid scopes, the cost is significantly less as well.

ENDOSCOPE HOLDERS

There are several types of endoscope holders available for neurosurgeons to use during endoscope procedures. Typically, the endoscope can be handled by the surgeon until reaching the desired location and angle of approach. Once the area of interest is reached, the endoscope can be locked in place, thereby freeing a hand and improving control. Flexible endoscopes must be placed in holders so that both hands can manipulate the control unit and the tip of the endoscope.

Semirigid Holders

Any of the flexible arms of the commonly available brain retractor systems can be adapted and used as an endoscope holder. For example, the flexible arm of the Leyla retractor (Integra, Plainsboro, NJ) can be attached to a rigid bar (Fig. 10) and be used as an adequate scope holder. The same can be done with the flexible arm of a Greenberg retractor (IM Greenberg, MD, Roslyn Estates, NY).

Rigid Articulated Nonpneumatic Holders

Storz manufactures an autoclavable endoscope system consisting of a socket clamp that attaches to the operating table, and articulated stand and a clamping jaw (Fig. 11). It is somewhat awkward to use and three points need to be loosened or tightened whenever an adjustment is necessary. However, it is very useful once the surgeon becomes used to using it.

Pneumatic Holder

Mitaka USA, Inc (Park City, UT) manufactures the Mitaka Point Setter pneumatic holding system, an OR table mounted holding system that holds a variety of surgical instruments including endoscopes. The system utilizes fail safe nitrogen breaks, and easily connects to hospital's operating room nitrogen systems. The holder's design allows for smooth surgeon control of the unit with joints that are designed for even movement with low friction (Figs. 12 and 13). The holder is designed for single hand

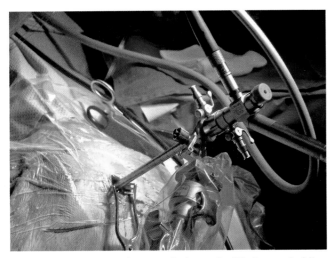

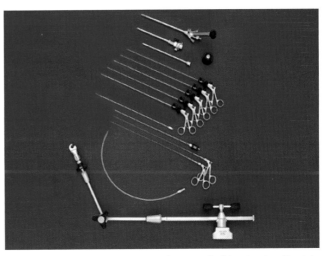

Fig. 10: Intraoperative photograph shows the Mitaka arm holding a rigid endoscope in place. The obturator metal sheet is seen in the burr hole and providing access to the ventricular system.

Fig. 11: The Storz semirigid endoscope holder is visualized in the lower most part of the photograph. Three joints with their appropriate tightening/loosening mechanism are illustrated.

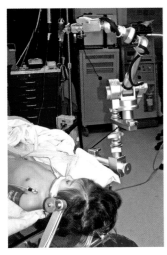

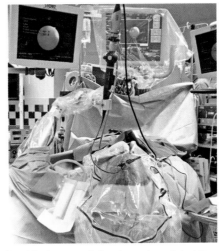

Fig. 12: The pneumatic Mitaka endoscope holder is seen attached to the bed before prepping and draping. Before starting the surgery, it should be properly positioned and secured so that it may reach the surgical field unhindered.

Fig. 13: The Mitaka arm fully draped and holding a flexible endoscope with the attached camera.

control and can be placed in many positions without backlash. This strong system is designed to hold heavy endoscopes with multiple instruments in a predictable and steady fashion. I have found it to be very versatile and reliable over many years.

ENDOSCOPIC INSTRUMENTS

Given the relatively small number of neuroendoscopic procedures performed (as compared to laparoscopic general, urologic, or gynecological procedures) the manufacturing companies have not developed as varied and extensive instrumentation for neurosurgery. Basically, instruments for both rigid and flexible scopes consist of only grasping and biopsy forceps as well as scissors and coagulators.

Biopsy Forceps

A pistol grip action allows for opening and closing the forcep's cups for tumor biopsy. Double action jaws allow for efficient tumor sampling (Figs. 14A to C). For rigid endoscopes semirigid forceps ranging from 1 mm to 2.3 mm and with working lengths of 30–45 cm are available for

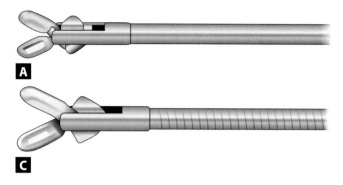

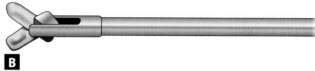

Figs. 14A to C: Different types of biopsy forceps. Typical size is 1 mm in diameter.

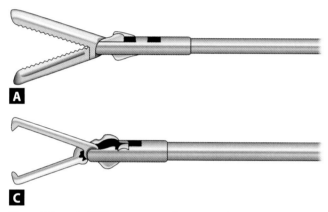

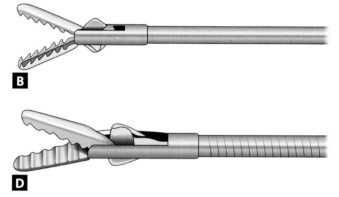

Figs. 15A to D: Different types of grasping forceps.

flexible endoscopes, flexible forceps of 1 mm diameter, and with a working length of 60 mm are also available.

Grasping Forceps

Often times, grasping cyst or tumor wall for endoscopic resection or mobilization is necessary. Grasping forceps are used and these single action instruments come both in flexible and semirigid forms to be used with flexible and rigid endoscopes, respectively. Likewise, they range in diameter from 1.0 mm to 2.3 mm and in working lengths between 30 cm and 60 cm (Figs. 15A to D).

Scissors

As with any other surgery, sharp dissection and cutting is performed in neuroendoscopic procedures miniature single or double action scissors are available for use. Introduced through the working channel, they vary in diameter between 10 mm and 2.7 mm and working lengths between 30 cm and 60 cm (Figs. 16A to D).

ELECTRODES

Monopolar

Achieving adequate hemostasis is extremely important in endoscopic surgery in a fluid medium. Any amount of blood in the fluid, no matter how small, will lead to a significant decrease in visualization. Consequently, obtaining hemostasis is virtually a necessity in order to perform these cases. Energy sources are needed to accomplish appropriate hemostasis and come in the mono- or bipolar variety. Several instrument sets come with these electrodes or they are available for third party vendors. A typical coagulating electrode attaches to a standard monopolar energy source, commonly available in all operating rooms such as the Codman's ME2 (microendoscopic electro) retractable monopolar system (Fig. 17) or Cook's monopolar electrode with ball tip or pencil point tip. Coagulation energy may also be delivered with bipolar electrodes as seen in Figure 18.

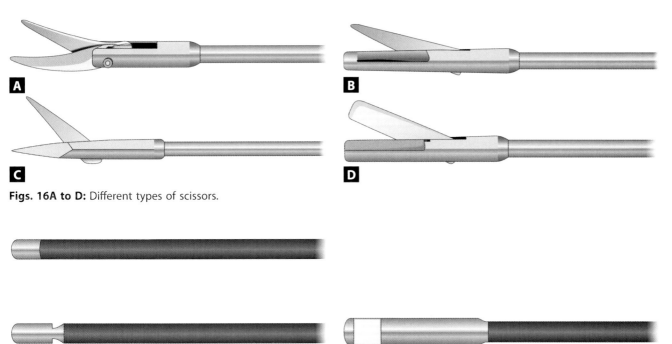

Figs. 16A to D: Different types of scissors.

Fig. 17: Different types of monopolar electrodes used through the endoscope's working channel..

Fig. 18: A bipolar electrode. Current moves between electrodes placed proximally and distally producing coagulating energy.

Lasers

Laser energy delivery systems are excellent modalities to deliver hemostatic energy in an aqueous environment. These are manufactured so that the energy can be delivered through very long, flexible fibers of varying diameters.

Nd:YAG Laser

Neodymium-doped yttrium-aluminum-garnet (Nd: YAG) is a crystal that is used as a source of providing energy for solid state lasers. Neodymium is used as the dopant for doping agent replaces small fraction of the yttrium and provides the lasing activity of the crystal. Nd:YAG lasers are optically pumped using laser diodes and emit light with a wavelength of 1,064 nm in the infrared spectrum. The laser light absorbs mostly in the bands between 730 nm and 760 nm, which is close to the absorption spectra of hemoglobin. This characteristic makes the Nd:YAG laser ideal for coagulation during neurosurgical procedures in the cerebrospinal fluid environment. The energy is delivered through long fibers of varying diameters (220 nm, 365 nm, or 550 nm) all which easily fit into the working channel of the endoscopes. Energy can vary between 1 watt to as high as 100 watts. Most of the work can be done within a range of 5–20 watts. The unit can be set to deliver single pulses or on a continuous mode. I found the Nd:YAG laser to be extremely versatile and useful when approaching a vascularized lesion (cyst wall, tumor capsule, etc.) the laser tip can be positioned at 5 mm or 10 mm from the target and as the energy is delivered, it diffuses and causes hemoglobin denaturing and the vessels disappear as if being painted with a white air brush. Once devascularized, the capsule can be opened with direct contact with the fiber. As such, it acts as a cutting tool as well (Fig. 19).

Potassium-Titanyl-Phosphate Laser

A potassium-titanyl-phosphate (KTP) crystal doubles the frequency of pulsed Nd:YAG laser to a 532 nm wavelength located in the green electromagnetic spectrum. It also absorbs hemoglobin in an excellent manner and obtains coagulation and is not absorbed by water. As with YAG lasers, the energy can be delivered via long fiber cables of varying diameters and can be placed inside the endoscope working channel.

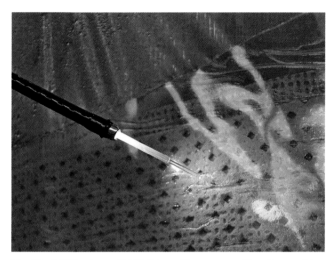

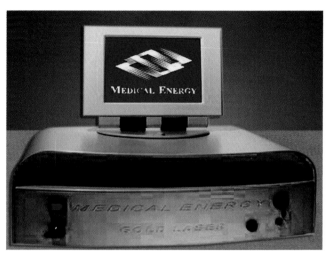

Fig. 19: A 535 micron Nd:YAG laser fiber seen exiting the working channel of a flexible endoscope. The red light indicates the location of where the energy will be delivered.

Fig. 20: GOLD LASER delivery system.

2 Micron Laser

The newest laser is available is the 2 micron laser, which is almost identical to the well-established Holmium laser. The laser offers the cutting an ablation properties of the CO_2 laser, the excellent hemostasis of the Nd:YAG laser, and the shallow tissue effect of Holmium lasers. The tissue effect or damage is restricted to less than 1 mm beneath the cut. Vision impairment is minimal as no or minimal bleeding is encountered. This color neutral laser does not produce a visible glare as with KTP lasers. A significant advantage of this laser is that it does not require special power outlets (a standard 100–240 VAC can be used) and no cooling water is necessary. Power to tissue can vary between 1 watt and 30 watts, has a repetition rate of 0.5–10 Hz, and an aiming beam of 635 nm (USA laser products OHG, Katlenburg-Lindau, Deutschland). I have been using this laser for the past several years with excellent results.

Gold Laser

L-F 20/30/40 Gold Laser, manufactured by Medical Energy, Inc. (Pensacola, FL) is a new type of laser that is perfectly suitable for neuroendoscopic procedures in an aqueous environment and with great coagulating capabilities. The GOLD LASER™ is a solid-state laser that operates in the infrared spectrum in the 980 nm to 1000 nm levels (Fig. 20). The laser can be used outside of the ventricular system using a hand held delivery system

(Fig. 21). This laser can be used in the continuous wave (CW) or pulsed wave (PW). It utilizes an active medium comprised of indium Gallium III Arsenide Phosphide (InGaAsP0 and the element gold (Au) both which emit energy in near infrared spectrum. This laser technology provides precise cutting, vaporization and coagulation simultaneously whilst controlling depth of penetration into the surrounding tissue, thus making it an ideal advanced tool for neuroendoscopic procedures. The LASERPOWERTOUCH Fiber Delivery Systems provides the surgeon with an array of different tip designs (Fig. 22). For instance, the angled, side firing, forward emission fiber delivery system is designed to deliver laser energy at 38 degrees. The Ball tip provides 360 degrees of contact surgical application, working only where tissue is touched. In **neurosurgical brain tissue procedures**, the laser gives the surgeon the ability to denature, vaporize, seal small bleeding vessels, and excise brain tumors, cysts, and scar tissue. The product offers a tangible technique, delivery through fluid, and precision contact and noncontact surgical application of less than < 0.3 mm while preserving surrounding healthy tissue and nerves.

Balloon Catheters

A very useful instrument in endoscopy is the balloon catheter. The balloon is located at the tip of a flexible catheter and inflates with air (Fig. 23). The typical

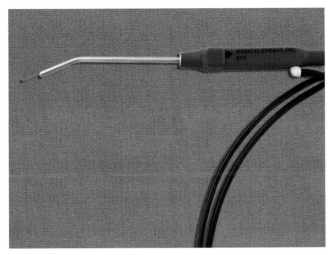

Fig. 21: Hand piece that can be used to deliver the GOLD LASER energy when not passing the laser fiber through the working channel of the endoscope.

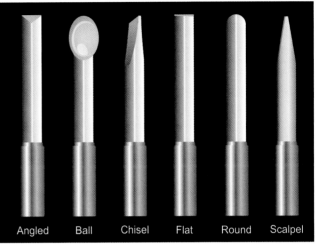

Angled Ball Chisel Flat Round Scalpel

Fig. 22: The above tip designs indicate the distal, working end of the LASERPOWERTOUCH™ Fiber Delivery Systems of the GOLD Laser technology.

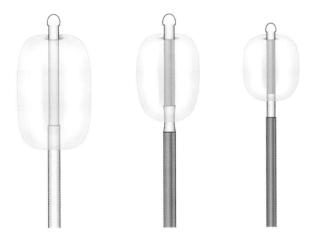

Fig. 23: Balloon catheters are very useful in neuroendoscopy. They are typically used to expand an ostomy or opening. Also may be used for tamponade bleeding.

3 French size allows the catheter to be deployed through the working channel. It is very useful for dilation of the fenestrated cyst wall or for opening an ostomy, as in the floor of the third ventricle. A relatively atraumatic method for expanding the opening, these catheters are very valuable in neuroendoscopy.

CONCLUSION

Although there is not a very extensive array of instrumentation available for neurosurgical procedures, what is available is sufficient to do the necessary work. As with all else, a good knowledge and understanding of the endoscopes and instruments will aid the surgeon in performing efficient and safe surgeries.

CHAPTER 4

Approaches to the Ventricular System

David F Jimenez

INTRODUCTION

This chapter details the best approaches to reach the human cerebral ventricular system using endoscopic techniques. The selection of proper entrance portals is extremely important for achieving a successful outcome and to minimize complications. Proper burr hole location and trajectory to specific lesions is described in detail. Access to the third ventricle as well as to the frontal, occipital and temporal horns is presented.

GENERAL PRINCIPLES

As with all neurosurgical procedures, the patients are given a single dose of intravenous antibiotics within 30 minutes of making a scalp incision. General anesthesia principles are used, as these cases require the patient be fully anesthetized. Position of the patient is dependent on the area to be accessed but most cases can be done in the supine position with the head rotated or angulated for best access. Proper scalp prepping is done with povidone-iodine solution. Care is taken to avoid the use of alcohol or alcohol-based solutions as there is a significant risk of fire if electrocautery is used with a scalp or hair wet with alcohol. It is of absolute importance as well, to make sure that all endoscopic equipment needed is in the room ready for use and properly sterilized. Equally important is the need to make sure that all of the endoscopic equipment is properly working, particularly the audio-visual system and monitors. The use of a surgeon's rolling stool with adjustable arm rests is also an imperative. By sitting and resting the elbows on the arm rests, the surgeon obtains superior hand stability and minimizes arm and hand fatigue (Fig. 1). Trying to do these surgeries while standing up will lead to rapid fatigue, tremors, and poor endoscopic control. The viewing television monitors must be set up in such a way that the surgeon faces them directly when operating. Having the monitors to the side will lead to cervical discomfort and neck fatigue (Fig. 2). The irrigant of choice is lactated ringers warmed to 37°C. The use of normal saline (average pH of 5.1) is contraindicated and has been associated with complications. The use of self-retaining endoscopic retractors is very useful in neuroendoscopy. Once the target area has been found, the endoscope can be set in a specific location, thereby freeing one of the surgeon's hands. A number of retractors

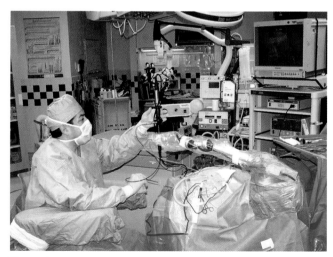

Fig. 1: Proper ergonomic OR set up: surgeon sits on surgical stool with padded arm rests set at appropriate height. Both hands are free to manipulate the endoscope and instruments. Both feet are also free to control the irrigation and laser/monopolar units.

can be used and range from adapting a ubiquitous Leyla brain or Greenberg retractor to a fully pneumatized and highly precise holder such as a Mitaka Point Setter arm (Mitaka USA Inc, Park City, Utah) (Figs. 3 to 5).

It is my preference to first access the ventricular system with a silastic ventricular catheter. This maneuver minimizes neural tissue damage while attempting to cannulate the ventricle, particularly when they are small. Additionally, the use of a manometer allows for measurement of intracranial pressure (ICP) and for testing of cerebral compliance, if so desired. For placement of the endoscope into the ventricular system, a port is used.

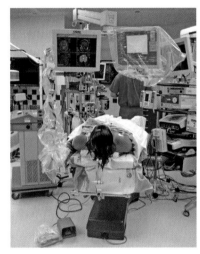

Fig. 2: The viewing monitors should be situated in a way that the surgeon, assistant and surgical technician can view them directly and without turning their heads during the case.

My preference is a disposable 14 French Peel-away introducer (Codman, Raynham, MA) (Fig. 6). This product allows for repeated endoscopic placement into the ventricles without causing repeated damage. Its diameter is larger than the endoscope and as such cerebrospinal fluid (CSF) and irrigation fluid escape passively. The introducer of the many endoscopic systems available come with their own built-in metal introducers which work very well. Prior to entering the ventricular system, the surgeon must make sure that the endoscope and TV image are properly and adequately aligned with the patient's head position. The best way to do this is to hold the endoscope at a distance far enough from the patient so that it matches the image on the monitor. The surgeon then moves the scope northward, south, east, and westward and the movements should match between the surgeon's hands and the TV monitor view. Failure to do so will lead to disorientation and possible injury to the patient.

FRONTAL HORN ACCESS

The frontal horn provides access to multiple areas of interest including the frontal horn itself, the septum pellucidum, the foramen of Monro, the anterior and posterior third ventricle as well as to the body of the lateral ventricle. However, in each case the frontal horn is accessed through a different angle of approach. In most cases the patient is positioned supine and with the head neutral or slightly flexed. Most commonly the head is placed in 3-point rigid fixation but a cerebellar horseshoe head holder may be

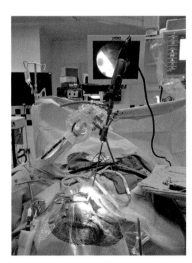

Fig. 3: A rigid endoscope, with its working channels (Oi system), properly set on a Mitaka holder. The holder can be pneumatically repositioned as the surgery progresses while allowing the surgeon to use both hands to handle the instruments.

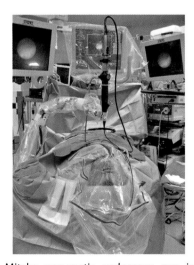

Fig. 4: The Mitaka pneumatic endoscope arm is very useful for holding the endoscopic system in place while performing surgery. Nitrogen driven and with multiple articulating joints, it provides an excellent range of reach and positions. Photograph shows draped holder with a flexible endoscope set in place.

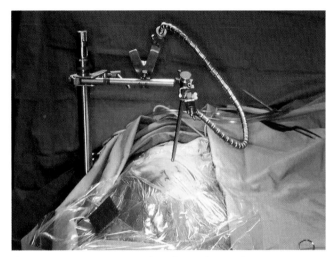

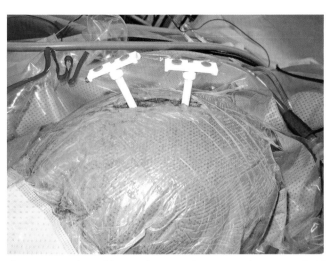

Fig. 5: A more economical and simpler endoscope retractor is obtained by adapting and using a flexible Leyla Retractor. Attached to a bed bar, it is seen here holding the metal introducer of the GAAB system.

Fig. 6: An ipsilateral biportal approach to an endoscopic colloid cyst resection. Note the lateral placement of the portals.

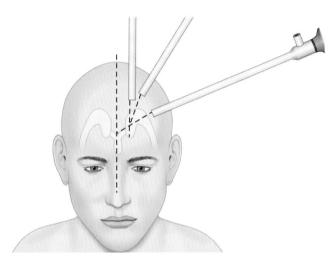

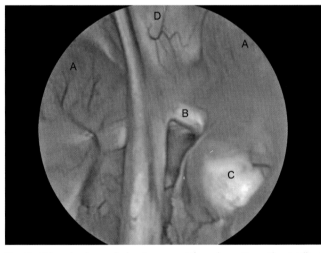

Fig. 7: Access to the frontal horn is gained via a frontal burr hole. However, the exact point of entrance will vary depending on the location of the lesion or target point.

Fig. 8: When hydrocephalus is present for a long time, the midline septum pellucidum disappears as seen in this image. Both frontal horns are seen with the genu and rostrum of the corpus callosum making the front and floor of the frontal horns, respectively. (A: Head of the caudate; B: Fornix; C: Thalamic tubercle; D: Genu of the corpus callosum).

used as well. Location of the entrance burr hole is made based on the MR images cross referencing all three planes (Fig. 7). If neuronavigation is available, then the entrance point should be precisely located in the operating room once the patient has been registered and the MR data entered into the work station. The standard frontal horn access point (Kocher's point) should not automatically be used (Fig. 8). For septum pellucidotomies, colloid cysts, and suprasellar arachnoid cysts, a far lateral

approach is needed (Figs. 9A and B). Additionally, the surgeon may choose to use a biportal technique (Figs. 10 and 11). For third ventriculostomies, the burr hole is placed behind the coronal suture (Fig. 12). This placement allows the scope to reach the foramen of Monro from a posterior approach and as the scope is advanced forward, it gains direct access to the tuber cinerium without placing any unnecessary pressure on the fornix. At the end of the procedure, a piece of Gelfoam®

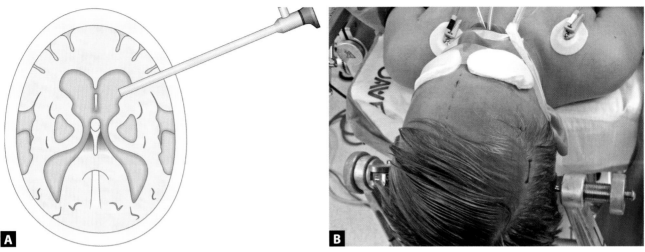

Figs. 9A and B: (A) Access to the frontal horn for performing a septum pellucidotomy requires that the burr hole be placed far lateral (up to 7 cm from midline) so that the septum may be visualized en-face. (B) Intraoperative photograph of patient undergoing a septum pellucidotomy. A far lateral portal has been selected.

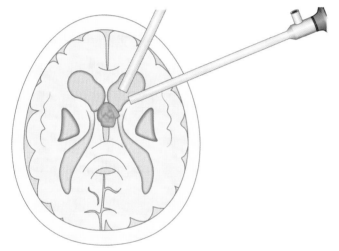

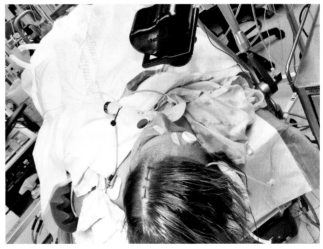

Fig. 10: Diagram showing a biportal approach for resection of a colloid cyst. One port is used to place the endoscope and the second port is used to introduce suction or other instruments. Such an approach increases the surgeon's flexibility in managing the lesion and its removal.

Fig. 11: Intraoperative photograph of a patient set up for a biportal endoscopic resection of a colloid cyst. The incisions are made lateral to Kocher's point and in front and behind the coronal suture.

(Pharmacia and Upjohn Co, Kalamazoo, MI) is inserted into the burr hole and a titanium burr hole cover plate is used to cover the opening. This maneuver prevents the scalp from sinking into the hole and causing pain and discomfort to the patient.

POSTERIOR THIRD VENTRICULAR ACCESS

For lesions located in the posterior third ventricle such as pineal region lesions, metastasis, tectal tumors, or membranes covering the aqueduct of Sylvius, an anterior frontal approach is preferred when using a rigid endoscope (Figs. 13A and B). The skin incision is made on the forehead along one of the natural forehead creases (Fig. 14). Once healed, the scar is barely visible. This approach allows the endoscope to enter the tip of the frontal horn (Fig. 15), and the foramen of Monro is directly visualized. Advancing the scope through the foramen of Monro and without placing any unnecessary torque on its structures, the posterior third ventricle can easily and rapidly be reached. The massa intermedia, connecting both thalami, posterior commissure, pineal recess, pineal gland region, aqueduct and posterior third ventricular wall are easily visualized (Fig. 16). If a flexible endoscope is used, a standard frontal horn access port may be used (Kocher's point) the endoscope is advanced through the foramen and then the tip is flexed posteriorly to reach the lesion (Fig. 17). However, the use of flexible endoscope requires considerable more experience and may be associated with more complications in the hands of an inexperienced endoscopist. Particularly difficult is the removal of the endoscope, as the surgeon can not see the

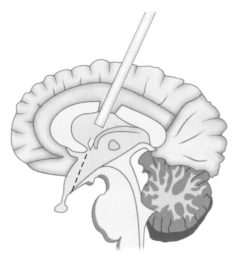

Fig. 12: Ideal placement of entry point for a third ventriculostomy places the burr hole behind the coronal suture so that the endoscope passes through the foramen of Monro and enters the anterior third ventricle.

structures behind the tip of the scope. For instance, simply pulling back an endoscope that has a flexed tip will cause damage to structures on its way out. The endoscope needs to be flexed and rotated simultaneously and when removing it, corrections need to be made. As the tip of the scope comes close to surrounding tissue, the light will bleach the tissue, indicating near or close contact with the tissue. As the scope is removed, small corrections are made with the goal of moving the bright area away from the scope's view, thereby deflecting the tip away from the ventricular walls, fornix, or other critical structures. Once finished, gelfoam and burr hole cover are used to cover the defect. Running nylon is used to close the scalp and prevent postoperative spinal fluid leaks.

ANTERIOR THIRD VENTRICULAR ACCESS

Access to the anterior third ventricle is most commonly done for third ventriculostomies but other lesions may present there such as cysts, tumors, hamartomas, or infections. The patient is placed supine and with slight extension. The placement of the burr hole is critical for an excellent result. The goal is to reach the ventricle and area of interest without placing any undue pressure or torque on the structures comprising the foramen of Monro. Consequently, the best place to locate the burr hole is approximately 2 cm behind the coronal suture and 3–4 cm from the midline (Fig. 18). The actual location should be obtained using triplanar MRI slices or, if available,

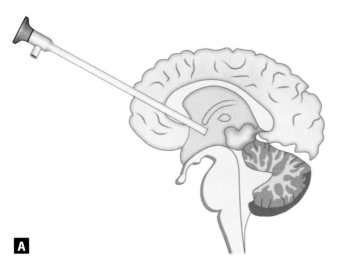

A

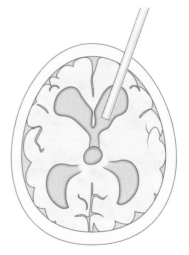

B

Figs. 13A and B: (A) For lesions located in the posterior third ventricle, an anterior frontal approach is necessary. The scalp incision is made along a forehead furrow and the tip of the frontal horn entered. Direct entrance into the posterior third ventricle is thus obtained. (B) An axial diagram showing the position of the endoscope for accessing a posterior third ventricular lesion.

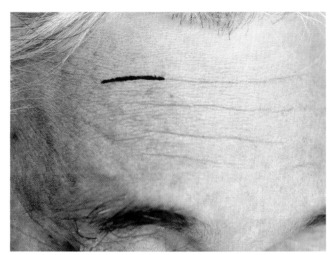

Fig. 14: The skin incision used to access lesions located in the posterior third ventricle. The incision is localized lateral to the mid-pupillary line and on a forehead crease, which allows for excellent scar healing and concealment.

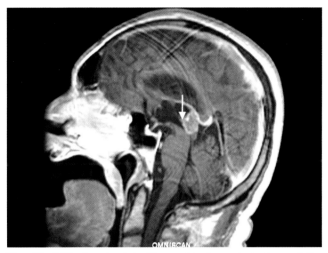

Fig. 15: MRI of patient in Figure 14 shows trajectory of the endoscope (white arrow) through the foramen of Monro to reach this third ventricular germinoma. If possible, as in this case, an ETV can be performed through the same portal. (ETV: Endoscopic third ventriculostomy).

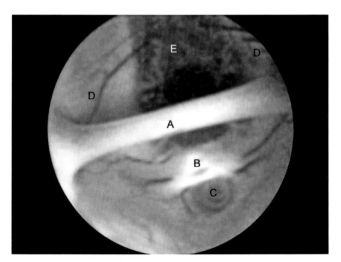

Fig. 16: Posterior third ventricle structures: (A) Massa intermedia; (B) Posterior commissure; (C) Aqueduct of Sylvius; (D) Thalami; (E) Tela choroidea and choroid plexus on the roof of the ventricle.

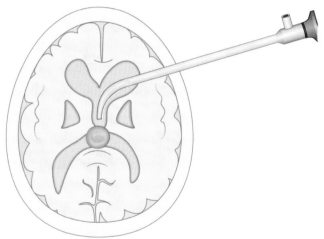

Fig. 17: A posterior third ventricular lesion can also be reached using a flexible endoscope through a standard frontal approach. This procedure requires a higher level of expertise and good knowledge of flexible scope dynamics.

neuronavigation. Once the ventricle is cannulated, the foramen will be visualized and the endoscope advanced into the third ventricle. The structures seen will include the mammillary bodies, tuber cinerium, infundibular recess (and its associated reddish color), optic chiasm, suprachiasmatic recess, lamina terminalis, and the anterior commissure (Figs. 19A and B). Once the procedure is finished, closure is done in the aforementioned fashion. A commonly encountered problem is a suprasellar arachnoid cyst that extends superiorly and elevates the third

ventricle and expands and blocks the foramen of Monro. A far lateral access is an excellent way to approach and fenestrate these lesions (Fig. 20).

OCCIPITAL HORN ACCESS

To access the occipital horn, trigone, or body of the lateral ventricle, the patient is positioned supine with a shoulder roll and the head turned to be parallel with the floor. Some surgeons place the patient prone or on a full

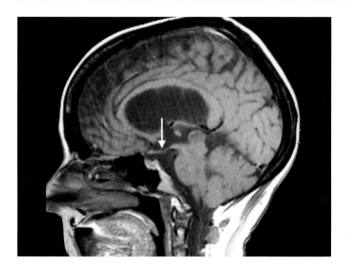

Fig. 18: Sagittal MRI shows location (white arrow) of where the ostomy is made in an ETV (endoscopic third ventriculostomy).

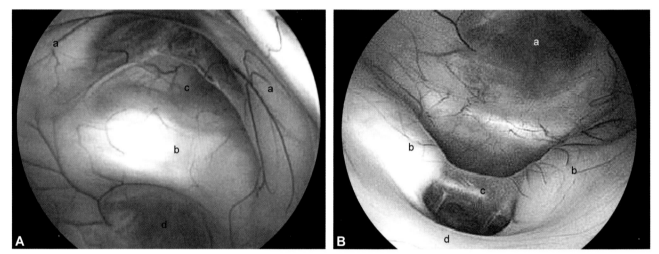

Figs. 19A and B: Anterior ventricular anatomy: (A) (a) Hypothalamic walls; (b) Optic chiasm; (c) Lamina terminalis; (d) Infindibular recess. (B) (a) Infindibular recess; (b) Mammillary bodies; (c) Basilar artery tip; (d) Mesencephalon.

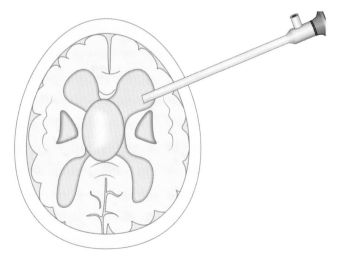

Fig. 20: Far lateral burr hole placement for accessing a large suprasellar arachnoid cyst through the foramen of Monro. The cyst can be fenestrated into the ventricle and if needed, the basal cisterns.

lateral decubitus position. Location of the burr hole is in the classical position for occipital access: 3 cm lateral to the inion and 6 cm or 7 cm superiorly (Fig. 21). The exact location however should be obtained with neuronavigation or using triplanar MR images. Once the introducer is inserted into the ventricle the endoscope is passed and the occipital horn is visualized. Structures seen in this area include the calcar avis, collateral trigone, choroid plexus, and posterior thalamus. Lesions encountered in this area include trapped cysts, meningiomas, metastasis, and neurocisticercosis.

FOURTH VENTRICULAR/ CEREBELLAR ACCESS

The patient may be placed lateral with the neck in maximum allowable flexion to gain better access. The side of

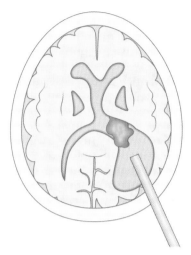

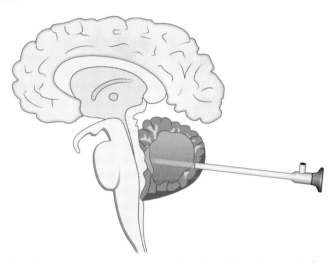

Fig. 21: Diagram showing the entrance point for a trigone-based lesion such as a meningioma. Entrance through a superior parietal lobule approach may suffice as well.

Fig. 22: A posterior fossa paramedian burr hole gains access for treating and fenestrating a trapped fourth ventricle.

the affected lesion should be above the horizontal plane. Lesions commonly encountered in this region include trapped fourth ventricle, arachnoid cysts, tumors, or neurocisticercosis. Even for midline lesions, the burr hole may be placed in a paramedian position. As with all other approaches, neuronavigation or MR images are used to select the best location for entrance. When operating on infants, care must be taken to avoid areas where large venous lakes are located such as the midline or at the level of the circular sinus. Once the endoscope is inserted and placed inside the trapped ventricle (Fig. 22), a fenestration can be done with a laser or a similar energy source system. Scalp and dural closure is done as previously described.

TEMPORAL HORN ACCESS

This is perhaps one of the least used approaches but may be encountered from time to time. The patient should be placed supine with an ipsilateral shoulder roll and contralateral head rotation. Entrance should be where the ventricle comes closes to the cortical surface, but most likely it should be about 1 cm above the ear. The middle temporal gyrus is the location of choice for the cortisectomy (Fig. 23). Most of the time the temporal horn is dilated and the ventricle is easily entered. Being that this is not a commonly entered area, the anatomy can be disorienting. Neuronavigation is of critical importance when working in this area. Nevertheless, choroid plexus can be used to help with localization. Remember that it

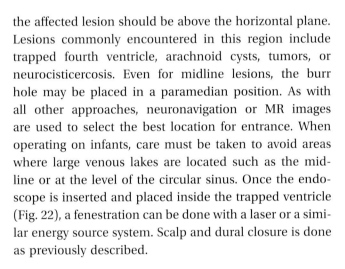

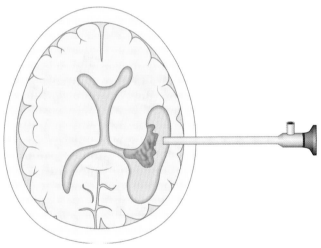

Fig. 23: Entrance into a trapped temporal horn with a lesion is achieved via a burr hole slightly superior to the pinna of the ear and through the middle temporal gyrus.

is located medially and superiorly when present in the temporal horn.

CONCLUSION

Choosing the appropriate angle of approach is of utmost importance for a successful endoscopic approach in the ventricular system. The principles described in this chapter should help the surgeon achieve a successful result. Failure to do so will place the patient at risk and increase the likelihood of complications.

CHAPTER 5

Third Ventriculostomy

David F Jimenez, David N Garza

INTRODUCTION

Treatment of hydrocephalus in modern times began almost 100 years ago with Dandy performing the first nonendoscopic third ventriculostomy in 1922 and Mixter the first endoscopic procedure in 1923. These procedures were mostly abandoned with the introduction of the ventricular shunts. Endoscopic third ventriculostomy (ETV) has had a significant resurgence in the recent decades. Nowadays, it is the preferred treatment method when a patient with non-communicating hydrocephalus presents to a pediatric neurosurgeon. It has also gained more acceptance in the adult neurosurgery community. The goal of this chapter is to present the history, indications and surgical technique for performing a third ventriculostomy.

PATHOLOGY AND CLASSIFICATION OF HYDROCEPHALUS

Hydrocephalus is a common condition in which infants and young children experience accelerated head growth caused by the accumulation of cerebrospinal fluid (CSF) in the skull. In adults, the clinical presentation includes chronic headaches, head pressure, imbalance as well as memory and cognitive problems. This accumulation is most frequently attributed to the inefficient absorption of CSF or some kind of physical obstruction. Cases in which the flow of CSF is physically hindered are classified as noncommunicating or obstructive; cases in which the flow is hindered by inefficient CSF absorption are classified as communicating or nonobstructive.[1] Obstructive cases include hydrocephalus secondary to congenital aqueductal stenosis or compressive (tectal or pineal tumors), tumors of brainstem, cerebellar infarct, Dandy-Walker malformation, encephalocele, intraventricular hematoma, colloid cysts, arachnoid cysts, amongst many causes.[2] Nonobstructive cases usually involve hydrocephalus secondary to intraventricular hemorrhage, ventriculitis, or meningitis. The incidence of pediatric hydrocephalus is about 1.1 per 1,000 infants.[3]

The traditional model used to explain the pathology of hydrocephalus is the "bulk flow" theory. Within that construct, intracranial pressure is said to be dependent on the balance maintained between the purported sites of CSF production (the choroid plexus) and absorption (the Pacchionian granulations or arachnoid villi). The theory has empirical roots that date back to 1914, when Dandy and Blackfan successfully produced hydrocephalus in a dog by obstructing its cerebral aqueduct.[4] Their findings contributed to the development of bulk flow theory and the concept of CSF malabsorption, but no one has ever been able to reproduce the observations made in that famous experiment.[5,6] Dandy himself explicitly discredited the bulk flow model in his writing. He objected to the idea that the Pacchionian granulations were solely responsible for absorption and suggested, instead, that CSF passes into the cerebral capillaries.[7] In 1910, even before Dandy and Blackfan's experiment, Mott proposed that it was possible for significant quantities of CSF to be resorbed into the bloodstream because brain capillaries were in communication with extracellular fluid spaces.[8] Contemporary evidence derived from radionucleotide cisternography and cardiac-gated magnetic resonance imaging (MRI) also challenges the validity of the bulk flow theory.[8,9]

Many authors recognize the need for theoretical revision and several support the notion that the cerebral capillaries play an integral role in CSF regulation.[5,6,9,10] Once CSF arrives at the capillary sites, it has been postulated that osmotic and hydrostatic forces regulate interstitial fluid (ISF) and CSF volume via fluid exchanges.[5] The notion that vascular forces are crucial to the maintenance of CSF circulation and changes in pulse pressure might incite communicating hydrocephalus was first suggested by O'Connell in 1943.[6,11] In 1997, Greitz et al. published a hypothesis building on these concepts later deemed the "hydrodynamic concept" of hydrocephalus. The model was grounded on the premise that CSF absorption occurs primarily through the capillaries and that communicating hydrocephalus was the result of increased arterial pressure.[9] The hydrodynamic concept divides hydrocephalus cases into two main groups: (1) acute hydrocephalus and (2) chronic hydrocephalus.[12] Acute hydrocephalus is effectively the same as noncommunicating hydrocephalus; it involves some sort of intraventricular CSF obstruction. Within the hydrodynamic concept, acute hydrocephalus is characterized by venous outflow compression with dilated capacitance vessels.[12]

Chronic hydrocephalus is organized into two subtypes: (1) communicating hydrocephalus and (2) chronic obstructive hydrocephalus.[12] The hydrodynamic theory does not ascribe CSF malabsorption to either subtype. Instead, it suggests that for chronic hydrocephalus patients ventricular enlargement can be attributed to the restricted expansion of the arteries and subsequent increase in capillary pulsations.[12] The increased systolic pressure distends the brain toward the skull and simultaneously compresses the periventricular region of the brain against the ventricles.[4] When the cerebral veins and capillaries become compressed, a significant reduction in blood volume occurs; this triggers a vicious cycle in which the narrow vessels and diminished blood volume cause intracranial compliance to further decrease and intracranial pulse pressure to further increase.[4,13]

During an ETV, surgeons fenestrate the third ventricle floor or the lamina terminalis in order to create a direct communication between the third ventricle and the extra-cerebral subarachnoid spaces.[14] Greitz writes that ETV alleviates hydrocephalus by venting ventricular CSF through the stoma, which reduces the systolic pressure. This also reduces the compression of the capacitance vessels, which restores some degree of venous compliance and further reduces the intracerebral pulse pressure.[4]

For chronic hydrocephalus patients, the primary goal of any treatment is not to increase the absorption of CSF, but to increase intracranial compliance.[12] For acute hydrocephalus patients, the goal is to decrease the size of the ventricles and reduce intracranial pressure by bypassing the intraventricular obstruction and reestablishing the flow of CSF from the ventricles to the subarachnoid space.[12] ETV is often considered the superior surgical approach to the treatment of hydrocephalus because it achieves these goals in a minimally invasive manner and avoids the long-term complications of other techniques, such as placement of a diverting shunt.

HISTORY OF ENDOSCOPIC THIRD VENTRICULOSTOMY

In 1922, Walter Dandy reported the first nonendoscopic ventriculostomy for the treatment of congenital hydrocephalus when he performed a fenestration of the lamina terminalis via a craniotomy using a transfrontal approach.[1] Dandy reasoned that in order to cure hydrocephalus, it would be necessary to drain the ventricular fluid into the subarachnoid spaces by puncturing the floor of the third ventricle.[15] Although the procedure had a high mortality rate, it still managed to arrest hydrocephalus in approximately 70% of the surviving patients.[16] The treatment was refined in 1923 when urologist William Mixter performed the first successful ETV using a cystoscope.[17] The procedure was technically difficult and the outcomes were not always ideal, but it was the only effective surgery available at the time. ETV eventually fell out of favor with neurosurgeons because ventriculoperitoneal shunt technology improved and boasted superior morbidity and mortality rates. Interest in ETV as a viable surgical option was finally rekindled after long-term results demonstrated that shunts actually have a high incidence of malfunction.[18] In the late 1980s ETV became more widespread when technological advancements to endoscopes and imaging tools made the procedure much easier to perform.[19] It was not until the 1990s, however, when Jones et al. reported a 50% shunt-free success rate (followed by 61% in 1994), that ETV finally began to enter mainstream surgical usage.[1] The technique finally started to shift from an acceptable alternative therapy to the treatment of choice for hydrocephalus cases induced by aqueductal stenosis.[19] Since that time, ETV has become one of the most performed and most reported neuroendoscopic procedures.

ETIOLOGIES OF HYDROCEPHALUS AND ASSOCIATED ENDOSCOPIC THIRD VENTRICULOSTOMY EFFICACY

It is not definitively clear if ETV is more effective than shunting at resolving hydrocephalus when the etiologies involve infection or hemorrhage, but many reports in the literature do indicate that ETV is a safe and effective treatment option for conditions that give rise to obstructive hydrocephalus.[20-22] Aqueductal stenosis is one such condition. It can be either congenital or acquired, but the acquired type has a better ETV success rate than the congenital form.[23] Clinical features of hydrocephalus caused by malformative aqueductal stenosis in the neonatal form are often typical; all infants without a previous history of intraventricular hemorrhage, prematurity, or neonatal meningitis who present with a rapidly increasing head circumference are suspect.[19] In the adolescent/adult onset form, a long clinical history, endocrine disturbances, Parinaud's sign, and associated type 1 neurofibromatosis can all be considered classic features.[19] According to a study conducted by Tisell et al. examining the effectiveness of ETV in treating noncommunicating hydrocephalus, only 50% of adult patients with primary aqueductal stenosis experienced long-term improvement.[24]

Patients with tumoral lesions located in the posterior fossa have a high incidence of hydrocephalus.[23] Several authors suggest that ETV be performed before tumor removal in order to alleviate intracranial hypertension and reduce the incidence of postoperative hydrocephalus.[25-27] Others believe the incidence of persistent hydrocephalus is too low to justify the routine use of preoperative ETV.[25] El Beltagy et al. have reported that the people who would most likely benefit from ETV before tumor surgery include those patients above 1.5 years of age, those without metastatic disease in the CSF, and those with totally excised gliomas and ependymomas rather than medulloblastomas.[25] In their study examining patients with obstructive hydrocephalus secondary to midline tumors (found in the midbrain, pontine, pineal, tectal plate, thalamic, and third ventricular regions), O'Brien et al. determined that single ETV had a long-term success rate of 68%; they found no significant relationship between tumor location and ETV success or failure.[28]

Ruggiero et al. argue that for the emergency control of hydrocephalus caused by posterior fossa tumors, ETV should be considered a suitable alternative to ventriculoperitoneal shunting and external ventricular drainage; it can quickly eliminate symptoms and, in doing so, prolong surgery scheduling.[26] During an endoscopic procedure, surgeons also have the opportunity to obtain a biopsy under direct vision. In their study examining patients with posterior third ventricle lesions and moderate to severe hydrocephalus, Roopesh et al. were able to achieve CSF diversion by third ventriculostomy and establish a histological diagnosis by taking a biopsy; the biopsy's high positive yield (100%) confirmed for the authors the superiority of ETV over other surgical approaches under these particular circumstances.[29]

Because of its minimally invasive nature and reduced risk for CNS infection, ETV has also been considered as a treatment for posthemorrhagic hydrocephalus.[23] Intraventricular hemorrhage in premature infants is one of the major causes of hydrocephalus in developed countries, affecting 15% to 20% of premature infants weighing less than 1,500 g at birth and almost 50% of infants weighing less than 750 g at birth.[30,31] Extensive studies examining the effects of ETV performed on intracranial hemorrhage patients are scarce, but the success rates available in the literature range from 37% to 60.9%.[20,31-33] Any preoperative ETV selection process would likely exclude posthemorrhagic hydrocephalus patients with distorted ventricular anatomy due to brain damage or poor surgical visibility due to the presence of intraventricular blood.[23] Ventricular dilation spontaneously resolves in approximately 65% of posthemorrhagic hydrocephalus cases involving premature infants.[19] For minor hemorrhages, the reabsorption of floating intraventricular clots permits the restoration of CSF circulation and the eventual resolution of ventricular dilation; in cases of severe hemorrhage (grade III or IV), the organization of Pacchionian granulations and netting of fibrin at the level of the subarachnoid spaces creates scars of fibrous tissue that might obstruct CSF pathways.[19] This can eventually induce chronic hydrocephalus and necessitate surgical intervention. Whether the origin of hydrocephalus is the result of intraventricular hemorrhage or infection, the mechanism ultimately responsible for causing hydrocephalus is the same. In both cases, the initiation of the inflammatory pathways can lead to the aforementioned intraventricular ependymal scarring.[34]

In the past, many studies concluded that ETV was characterized by a high failure rate when used to treat posthemorrhagic or postinfectious patients.[19,32,35,36] Other studies, particularly contemporary ones, have demonstrated more promising results. Siomin et al. reported that ETV is highly successful in posthemorrhage patients who have previously undergone shunt placement, particularly preterm infants.[32] Rates of ETV success for postinfectious hydrocephalus patients are comparable to those seen in posthemorrhagic patients. Siomin et al. reported a success rate of 64.3% for the postinfectious population portion of their study, Warf reported an overall success rate of 64%, and Zandian et al. reported a 54% success rate.[20,32,37] If it were coupled with the early extraction of parasites, ETV could be used to treat chronic, postinfectious hydrocephalus without evidence of outlet obstruction (as in postmeningitis, ventricular enlargement, or neurocysticercosis cases).[23] However, age must also be taken into consideration. Patients with postinfectious hydrocephalus who are younger than 2 years of age, have ETV success rates that are often 50% or less.[23] The reason for those low rates might have something to do with the cisternal scarring that frequently occurs in postinfectious cases; the presence of that scarring more than doubles the risk of ETV failure.[38]

ENDOSCOPIC THIRD VENTRICULOSTOMY AND SHUNT IMPLANTATION

Shunt implantation is a common treatment for hydrocephalus, but authors estimate that it can lead to complications in around 44.3% of cases during the first postoperative year; these often involve shunt fracture, shunt obstruction, and infection.[39] There is evidence that suggests shunting might also be associated with seizures. In a study conducted by Chadduck and Adametz, 22% of patients who required at least one modification for shunt malfunction had seizures and patients with a history of shunt infection had a 47% increased risk for developing seizures.[40] Shunt infection has been associated with neurological disability, reduced intellectual performance, and almost a twofold increase in long-term mortality rates.[41-44] Frequently, patients must undergo multiple visitations to manage the complications related to shunt placement. With ETV, there is a diminished concern for postoperative infection and no need to worry about malfunction or dependence. Shunt independence is especially important for patients living in developing countries who may not have immediate access to reliable health care professionals in the event of a shunt-related emergency. ETV is often the preferred initial approach to hydrocephalus treatment because it is minimally invasive

and typically involves shorter operative and recovery times, but ETV should not be understood exclusively as an alternative to shunting. For many patients who experience shunt-related complications, ETV can be used as a complementary approach to shunt treatment.

Originally, previously shunted patients were considered poor candidates for ETV because shunt therapy was thought to impair the mechanisms of CSF absorption. ETV was performed only in extremely complicated cases that required shunt removal, such as those involving recurrent blockage, infection, or slit ventricle syndrome.[45-48] However, those surgical outcomes were so encouraging that physicians started to expand the application of ETV to include all patients with shunt malfunction who presented with compatible anatomy.[45] The mindset that maintained shunt dependence as an absolute inevitability—"once a shunt, always a shunt"—slowly became dispelled. During the late nineties and early twenties, many experts assumed that patients with a history of CSF infection or hemorrhage were predisposed to ETV treatment failure.[32,25,36,49] However, a growing body of evidence was emerging that suggested whatever the etiology, there was a 50% to 70% chance third ventriculostomy would successfully cure hydrocephalus in previously shunted patients.[19,46,50] Subsequent studies have attempted to elucidate how precisely hydrocephalus etiology and shunt history affect a patient's surgical outcome. Whether ETV is used as the primary approach to treating hydrocephalus or as a secondary approach after shunt failure, the rates of success appear to be comparable. In their study examining both populations, O'Brien et al. reported that 74% of patients in their primary ETV group (126 out of 170) and 70% of patients in their secondary ETV group (44 out of 63) had successful surgical outcomes.[21] While the order of intervention alone did not appear to significantly impact surgical outcome, there were some noticeable differences in ETV success rates when the etiology of the patients' hydrocephalus was also taken into consideration. In O'Brien's primary ETV group, patients with a history of hydrocephalus due to intraventricular hemorrhage and meningitis had poor ETV success rates (27% and 0%, respectively). Within that group, the cases who predominately had successful outcomes were those involving spina bifida (88%), aqueductal stenosis (69%), and arachnoid cysts (100%). In the secondary ETV group, patients with hydrocephalus due to intraventricular hemorrhage and meningitis had success rates of 71% and 75%, respectively.[21]

O'Brien's findings affirm some of the observations reported in an earlier multicenter retrospective study conducted by Siomin et al. In 2002, those authors noted a high rate of success for ETV under two specific circumstances: (1) initial ETV that was used to treat hydrocephalus cases caused by primary aqueductal stenosis and (2) secondary ETV that was used to treat hydrocephalus cases caused by intraventricular hemorrhage that had previously undergone shunt placement.[21,32] It seems reasonable to conclude then that ETV is not often the best initial treatment for patients suffering from hydrocephalus caused by intraventricular hemorrhage or infection. ETV will more likely be effective as the initial treatment for obstructive hydrocephalus or as a secondary treatment approach for hydrocephalus cases caused by hemorrhage or infection that have been unsuccessfully treated with shunt placement.

FACTORS AFFECTING ENDOSCOPIC THIRD VENTRICULOSTOMY PATIENT OUTCOMES

Age is a major factor in determining the outcome of ETV surgery for hydrocephalus patients. While outcomes for patients older than 6 months are generally favorable, patients younger than 6 months have surgery success rates that range between 34.8% and 67%.[51-55] Ogiwara et al. report a success rate of 25% for obstructive hydrocephalus patients younger than 3 months of age.[54] Regardless of etiological factors, the impact of age on ETV failure seems to be most critical for infants within the first 2 months of life.[55] Some authors are less reluctant than others about performing ETV on younger patients, but most agree that it is still necessary to look at all other relevant variables before making a final decision regarding treatment. ETV failure usually occurs during the first few months after surgery, but there have been some reported cases of delayed failure. Rivero-Garvia et al. have suggested that moderate cranial growth restriction through the application of a fabric adhesive bandage might increase the success rate of ventriculostomies performed in patients less than 1 month of age when worn after surgery.[51] In the event of surgical failure, it is generally advisable to repeat the ETV procedure, especially if the first attempt was initially successful for an extended period of time.[23]

Patients who have shunt placement prior to undergoing endoscopic cyst fenestration require additional surgical intervention with more frequency than patients who have not experienced shunting. In a study conducted by Lewis et al., 6 out of 12 previously shunted hydrocephalus patients (50%) required another endoscopic cyst fenestration; only two of 22 patients without shunts (9%) required additional surgical intervention.[56] A study conducted by El-Ghandour yielded similar results. All hydrocephalus patients who had previously undergone shunt treatment required repeated endoscopic cyst fenestration; none of those patients were ever able to become shunt-independent because of the postoperative gliosis induced by previous shunt infection.[57] In a collaborative, multicenter international study conducted by Kulkarni et al., the authors determined that the deleterious impact of previous shunting experience on ETV success appeared to diminish in magnitude when compared to the favorable odds conferred by advanced patient age, the strongest predictor of ETV success.[58]

ENDOSCOPIC THIRD VENTRICULOSTOMY AND CHOROID PLEXUS CAUTERIZATION

It was once thought that a deficiency in CSF absorption contributed to ETV failure in infant populations. In the past, many physicians advocated performing choroid plexus surgery in conjunction with ETV in order to address that specific issue.[59] The technique started as early as 1910, when Lespinasse used a cystoscope to fulgurate the choroid plexus of two infants with hydrocephalus.[17] Dandy, however, is often credited as being the first person to formally propose the notion of treating nonobstructive hydrocephalus via choroid plexus excision in 1918.[15,60] He attempted to perform an endoscopic choroid plexectomy in 1922 but was ultimately unsuccessful; he finally removed a choroid plexus using a cystoscope in 1932 with results that were comparable to those of a formal craniotomy.[17] In 1934, Putnam reported on the effectiveness of cauterizing the choroid plexus with a ventriculoscope in order to treat hydrocephalus.[17,61] In 1936, Scarff developed an endoscope with several important enhancements, including: a lighting system, a "fore-oblique" lens-system that provided a wide angle, a movable electrode designed to facilitate cauterization, and an irrigation system that could clear away blood from the operative fiend and continuously replace any fluid escaping from the ventricles.[15,17,62] Scarff criticized Dandy's original technique because it emptied all the CSF from both ventricles before destroying the choroid plexus.[62] He noticed that draining the CSF predisposed the walls of the ventricles to collapse, which could bring about severe shock. Endoscopic cauterization was a significant advancement in the treatment of nonobstructive hydrocephalus because it enabled a surgeon to destroy the choroid plexus with a minimal loss of CSF, which minimized the threat of ventricular collapse and subsequent surgical shock.[62] Up until the 1940s, choroid plexus cauterization (CPC) was frequently used in the treatment of hydrocephalus; however, upon review, it was determined that the majority of patients undergoing the technique demonstrated progressive ventricular enlargement at a rate that was comparable to or greater than the preoperative rate.[16] As the years passed, interest in CPC began to wane. It was almost completely abandoned as a viable surgical technique in the 1970s, when Milhorat conducted a series of studies questioning its efficacy. In those experiments, Rhesus monkeys showed only a 40% decrease in CSF production after bilateral choroid plexectomy and a human patient who had undergone the same procedure had a normal rate of CSF production 5 years after surgery.[63] These findings, along with advances made in the development of valve regulation and biocompatible synthetic materials, encouraged most surgeons to adopt shunt placement as the superior treatment modality for hydrocephalus.[16] However, shunting eventually fell out of favor with physicians when they observed the long-term complications related to infection and mechanical malfunction; meanwhile, technology improved and made the neuroendoscopic approach more effective and safer to perform.

Choroid plexus cauterization was revisited as a viable procedure in 1995 when Pople and Ettles demonstrated how successful the technique could be under certain conditions. For children who had communicating hydrocephalus and a slow to moderate rate of increase in head circumference, they reported a 64% success rate; patients who presented with tense fontanels and rapidly progressive hydrocephalus had the lowest rate of success (around 12.5%).[63] The reason for this difference likely had something to do with one of the supposed limitations of endoscopic surgery. When CPC is performed endoscopically, many surgeons are capable of achieving only a partial coagulation of the choroid plexus. The residual choroid plexus located in the temporal horn continues producing CSF after surgery, so it has the potential to compensate for the change in CSF production attributed to

coagulation.[64] The slow progression of hydrocephalus in a patient suggests that he or she possesses a choroid plexus with limited function; under those conditions, CPC has a greater chance of contributing to overall surgical success.[64] Although some authors suggest that complete coagulation is impossible to achieve, Warf and Campbell have indicated that using a single endoscopic approach to cauterize the choroid plexus in both ventricles, including the temporal horns, is a feasible goal that can be mastered with practice, even by those surgeons who have no previous experience with ventriculoscopy.[65]

In 2005, Warf published a report in which he compared ETV performed by itself to ETV performed in conjunction with the neuroendoscopic cauterization of the choroid plexus. ETV's success rate increased from 47% (when performed alone) to 66% (after it was combined with CPC).[59] Warf determined that the combination of the two procedures was a superior treatment approach for infants younger than 1 year of age, particularly among those who had myelomeningocele and hydrocephalus that was not the result of infection.[59] Warf's 2005 report collected data from patients who were treated at the CURE Children's Hospital of Uganda. In 2014, he collaborated with Stone and conducted a prospective ETV study using a small North American patient population. The authors considered their new overall success rate of ETV performed in conjunction with CPC (59%) to be comparable to the overall success rate attained in the Uganda series, which suggested to them that more than half of all infants presenting with hydrocephalus can initially and successfully be treated using this combination approach.[34]

While having similar overall success rates is certainly significant, it should be noted that each study's patient population had a different etiology that was primarily responsible for inciting hydrocephalus within their respective communities. In Uganda and other developing countries, posthemorrhagic hydrocephalus in premature infants is rarely seen because infants with low birth weights generally do not survive; in the United States and other developed nations, posthemorrhagic cases are seen with much more frequency.[14] Because the socioeconomic disparity between these populations contributes so greatly to the etiological composition of their reported hydrocephalus cases, Warf et al. describe postinfectious and posthemorrhagic hydrocephalus as diseases of "poverty" and "prosperity", respectively.[14] ETV has captivated the attention of many physicians because it offers a potentially permanent solution to hydrocephalus without the long-term complications that accompany other therapies. For this reason, it is especially attractive as a treatment option for communities who have limited access to health care resources.[37] CPC has been described as a technique that helps "level the playing field" for ETV performed among patients of various ages who suffer from hydrocephalus caused by a range of etiologies.[34] However, based on the results of their joint study, Stone and Warf do not recommend the combined ETV/CPC approach for postmeningitic hydrocephalus cases in their North American practice; for postmeningitic cases, they believe that expectations regarding surgical outcome must be "tempered".[34]

Several other factors that seem to be relevant to the success of ETV/CPC include: the characterization of the patient's hydrocephalus, the presence or thickness of a septum pellucidum, patient age, and the quality of the prepontine cistern. Patients with severe forms of hydrocephalus (such as hydranencephalic hydrocephalus) that display a slow progression seem to make ideal candidates.[64] The absence of a septum pellucidum (or the presence of a thin septum) facilitates the intraoperative visibility and technical execution of a parietal approach to the bilateral choroid plexus.[64] With regard to age, evidence has demonstrated that ETV/CPC is more successful than ETV alone specifically when the approach is performed on infants younger than 1 year (particularly those with who have a nonpost infectious hydrocephalus etiology or myelomeningocele).[59] Maturation is possibly a relevant factor to surgical success because younger patients may not have the necessary anatomical development to accommodate the new efflux of CSF that arrives via the ETV stoma.[65] It has been suggested that the arachnoid granulations (Pacchionian bodies) play some role in CSF absorption; they emerge before birth as microscopic villi but do not appear to function in the absorption of CSF until later in life, once a child reaches toddler age (around 12 months).[66,67] It is possible that younger ETV patients benefit from CPC because the procedure helps compensate for an infant's diminished CSF absorption capabilities.

In a study examining predominately postinfectious hydrocephalus cases, Warf and Kulkarni determined that prepontine cistern scarring more than doubled the risk of ETV failure.[38] This tendency does not appear to be dependent on the etiology of a patient's hydrocephalus.

Preliminary data collected by Warf, Campbell, and Riddle suggests that for posthemorrhagic cases with open cisterns ETV/CPC is more likely to succeed; for posthemorrhagic cases with scarred cisterns, they are more likely to fail.[14] The status of a patient's aqueduct might also have some bearing on surgical outcome. In the study conducted by Warf and Kulkarni, the authors indicated that an open aqueduct increased the risk of failure by 50%.[38] Warf previously observed that 83% of patients who demonstrated an enlarged fourth ventricle also had an open aqueduct.[37] By using cranial ultrasonography to assess the size of the fourth ventricle, a physician might be able to better predict a patient's aqueductal patency and, by extension, his or her surgical outcome.

There are some authors who are suspicious of the purported benefits of CPC. They believe that because evidence has emerged demonstrating that the choroid plexus is not the sole site of CSF production, the efficacy of the technique in the treatment of hydrocephalus is questionable.[5] Because we are still exploring the nature of CSF formation/absorption and the precise role it plays in the pathology of hydrocephalus, more research must be done before any definitive conclusions can be reached.

SURGICAL PROCEDURE

Preoperative Preparation

Medical management of the patient is as previously described prior to surgery for endoscopic procedures and in particular, for ETV, proper burr hole placement is of utmost importance for a successful outcome. Basic anatomical knowledge points to the fact the tuber cinerium is located anterior to the foramen magnum and, consequently, the standard, Kochker's point burr hole placement is not ideal. The burr hole should be placed posteriorly and behind the coronal suture. The exact position can be triangulated simply on a preoperative MRI and using all three planes: (1) sagittal, (2) axial, and (3) coronal. If image guidance is available (which may not be in most developing countries), then the MRI data can be loaded into the image guidance station and the proper point selected. The ultimate goal is to have straight and direct access to the anterior third ventricle's floor without the need to angulate or torque the endoscope (Fig. 1).

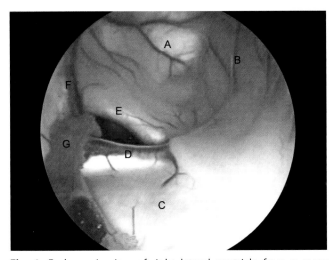

Fig. 1: Endoscopic view of right lateral ventricle from a more posterior approach shows a direct trajectory to the anterior third ventricle. The genu of the corpus callosum (A); head of the caudate (B); anterior thalamic tubercle (C); thalamostriate vein (D); fornix (E); septal vein (F); and choroid plexus (G) are clearly identified.

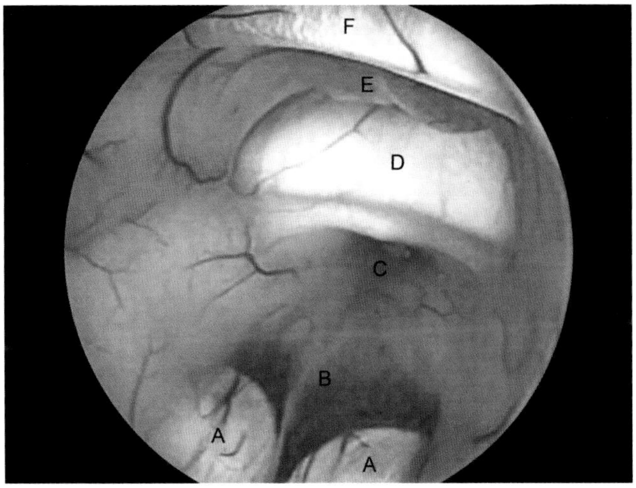

Fig. 2: Same patient as Figure 1. A direct view of the floor of the anterior third ventricle is seen as the foramen of Monro is traversed. Landmarks include: (A) mammillary bodies; (B) tuber cinerium; (C) infundibular recess; (D) optic chiasm; (E) lamina terminalis; and (F) anterior commissure.

Patient Positioning

This step is relatively straightforward as the patient is placed supine in a relatively neutral position. The patient can be placed on a horseshoe head holder or secured in pins with a Mayfield head holder. My personal preference is to use the latter for full security of patient's head as any movement during critical part of the procedure (when the anesthetic levels inadvertently drop and patient begins to move) could have catastrophic consequences. The surgeon's comfort is very important, and as such, I sit down for this procedure. I use a moveable Stryker stool with adjustable arms which can be set to have the surgeon's elbows close to 90°. This allows the surgeon to rest the elbows on the arm rest and minimize fatigue and tremor. Typically, the entire table needs to be placed at the lowest level so the head is in proper position in relation to the sitting surgeon's hands.

Burr Hole and Dural Opening

A standard burr opening is made with whatever tools are available to the surgeon (craniotome, drill tips, or even Hudson drill). The craniotome bit (ACRA-CUT®) leaves a circular rim of bone at the bottom of the hole, which can be removed with Kerrison Rongeours. This simple maneuver increases the working space at the dural level. For dural opening, my preference is to use a needle tip

monopolar set at 15 watts and create a cruciate opening in a bloodless fashion.

Ventricular Access

Once the proper trajectory to the ventricle has been selected, access can be achieved with a number of commercially available devices. I like to record the patient's intracranial pressure (ICP) prior to performing the procedure. This can be done by first placing a ventricular catheter into the ventricle and measuring ICP with a monometer. Most endoscopic systems come equipped with their own ventricular introducers. The introducer is passed into the ventricle to appropriate depth. The obturator is removed and the endoscope introduced into the ventricle. An alternate method (my preferred) is to use a disposable 14 French peel-away introducer (Codman, Rayham, MA) cut to a length of 10 cm. Likewise, it is passed forward and once the ventricle is cannulated, CSF can be seen at the center opening of the obturator, which is removed. The endoscope of choice is advanced and the lateral ventricle visualized. As the endoscope is passed through the foramen of Monro, the classical anatomy of the anterior third ventricle can be observed (Fig. 2).

The site of the ventriculostomy should be selected anterior to the mammillary bodies and posterior to the infundibular recess. The location should be midline, as

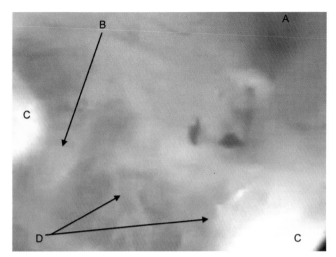

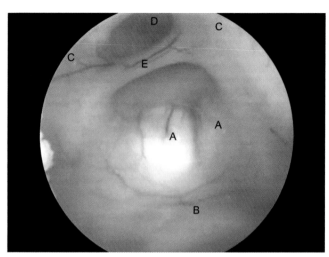

Fig. 3: Care must be taken to place the ostomy in the midline and immediately behind the infundibular recess (A). In this patient, the tuber cinerium is thin and transparent allowing visualization of the left oculomotor nerve (B) and basilar perforating vessels (D) as well as the mammillary bodies (C).

Fig. 4: Occasionally, the procedure will be more difficult by the presence of an interhypothalamic connection (E) extending from the medial hypothalamic walls (C); the infundibular recess (D); mammillary bodies (A); and mesencephalon (B) are easily identified.

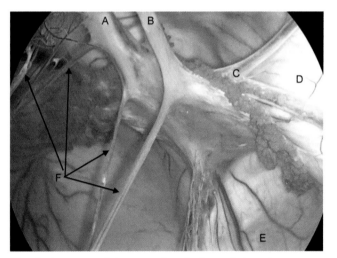

Fig. 5: In cases of longstanding hydrocephalus, the septum pellucidum disintegrate leaving only septal veins (F) the remaining fornix (A: left, B: right) are seen in a fully stretched state. The thalamostriate vein (C); anterior thalamic tubercle (D); and right calcar avis (E) are visible and identified.

place and both ventricles may be simultaneously visualized. The most important landmark is the choroid plexus, which when followed, will lead to the foramen of Monro. Once the foramen is transversed with the endoscope, access to the third ventricle is attained. If the burr hole has been properly placed there should be direct access to the floor of the anterior third ventricle. As the endoscope is passed through the foramen, the mesencephalon, mammillary bodies, and tuber cinerium should be clearly seen. The infundibular recess along with a group of hyper pigmented reddish cells should also be evident (Fig. 6). Preoperative MRI images should provide the surgeon with a clue as to the location of the basilar artery tip and its relation to the mammillary bodies.

Ventriculostomy Technique

The basic principle is to create an opening that communicates the third ventricle (and the rest of the ventricular system) with the basal cisterns. Much debate has occurred as to which is the best method to do so. Some authors prefer and recommend blunt puncture of the floor of the third ventricle with either a blunt probe or the endoscope itself (Fig. 7). That maneuver can be difficult to do particularly when the patient has a large ventricle and a stretched and patulous floor. In those cases, the floor moves along with the probe toward the basilar artery. Nevertheless, many authors have used the blunt

lateral placement significantly increases the risk of oculomotor nerve damage or injury to the medial hypothalamus (Fig. 3). Depending on the etiology and duration of the hydrocephalus, the patients' anatomy can vary significantly (Fig. 4). With longstanding hydrocephalus, it is not uncommon to see dissolution of the septum pellucidum (Fig. 5). In these cases only thin septal veins remain in its

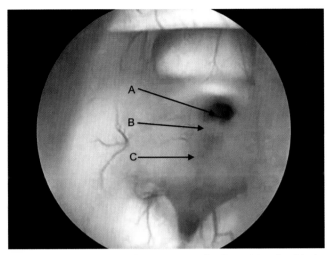

Fig. 6: Endoscopic view of third ventricular floor: (A) Infundibular recess; (B) hyper pigmented area where oxytocin and vasopressin are made; and (C) location of ventriculostomy.

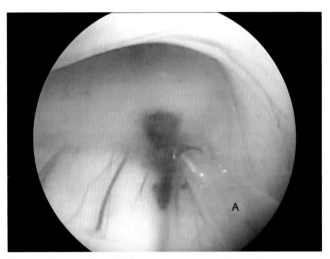

Fig. 7: Blunt probe (A) being used to mechanically open the ventricular floor often leads to small amounts of bleeding. Using an energy source minimizes bleeding.

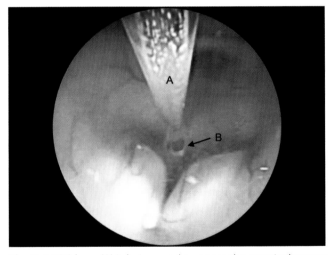

Fig. 8: A YAG laser (A) is being used to create the ventriculostomy (B). A red aiming beam is seen near the ostomy. The laser should be set at low wattage (2–3 watts).

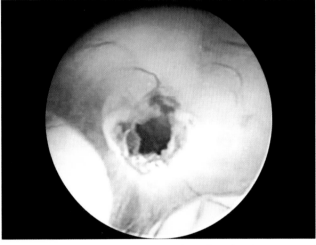

Fig. 9: The superficial most aspect of the floor has been opened with the laser and edges are cauterized.

technique with long lasting success. Another option is to use an energy delivery source to create the opening. A Bugby wire, a monopolar probe, or a laser fiber can all be used for this purpose. The key to a successful and safe ventriculostomy is to set the energy delivery source at a very low setting. My method of preference is to use a YAG fiber (100–600 microns) set at 2–5 watts and gently touch the floor on the selected area. As the energy is delivered, the tissue is cauterized and devascularized (Fig. 8). Irrigation of lactated ringers helps with further developing the opening (Fig. 9). Because the heat and energy produced by these devices extend to the surrounding tissues, and structures, there is significant concern that their use may lead to basilar artery injury. Lowering the amount of energy decreases the risk. Nevertheless, much care must be taken and perhaps should only be used by experienced endoscopists.

Once the opening has been made and close up view shows basal cisterns, it may be expanded with an expandable balloon such as a 3 French Fogarty catheter (Fig. 10). Various sizes and shapes are available to slowly and gently expand the opening (Fig. 11). The adequate

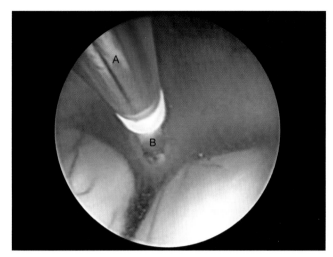

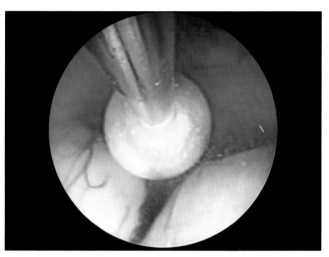

Fig. 10: Once the opening has been made, it is further expanded with the use of an expandable balloon catheter. The shaft (A) and collapsed balloon (B) are seen.

Fig. 11: The balloon has been fully inflated and the edges of the ventriculostomy are expanded thereby enlarging the opening.

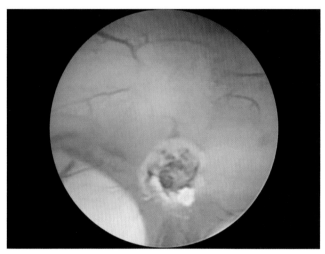

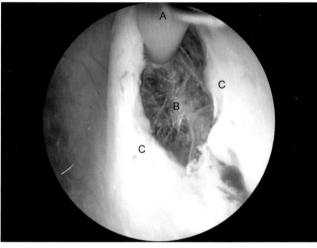

Fig. 12: A complete opening has been made and the third ventricle is in communication with the basal cisterns through the floor opening.

Fig. 13: Arachnoidal trabeculations (B) are seen beyond the opened ventricular floor (C). The laser fiber (A) can be used to mechanically expand the opening.

size of the ostomy is not known but it should be at least the size of the aqueduct of the Sylvius (2 mm). Most often an opening of 4–5 mm can be easily created. With true obstructive hydrocephalus, the flow of fluid should be from ventricle to cistern with every systole/diastole cycle, thereby keeping the opening patent. After the ostomy is made inspection of the basal interpeduncular cistern should be carefully undertaken (Fig. 12). Multiple arachnoid trabeculations are commonly seen (Fig. 13) as well as a prominent membrane of Liliequist (Fig. 14). Further opening of these trabeculations and membranes

should be carefully done to assure maximum success (Fig. 15). The trunk of the basilar artery and its perforating vessels can be seen (Fig. 16). Closure is done by removal of all instruments and access port. If desired, an external ventricular drain may be left overnight to monitor ICP and then remove it the following day. The burr hole is covered with a burr hole plate and the scalp closed with two layers: (1) absorbable galeal suture and (2) nonabsorbable dermal suture. Most patients can be discharged the following day, if an uneventful procedure has taken place.

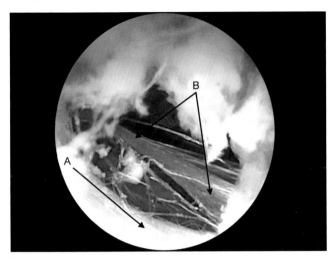

Fig. 14: Closer view of the ventriculostomy reveals the membrane of Liliequist (B) as well as the top of the basilar artery (A).

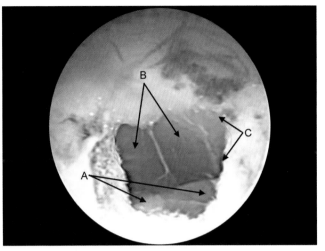

Fig. 15: After successful ventriculostomy is done, the open basal cistern is seen along with the top of the basilar artery (A); edges of the resected tuber cinerium (C); and the clivus (B).

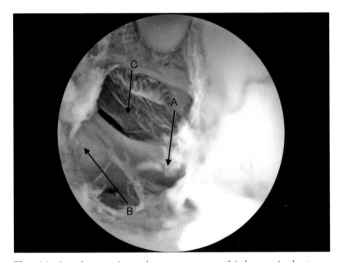

Fig. 16: Another patient shows a patent third ventriculostomy and the basilar tip (A), P1 segment of the posterior cerebral artery (B); and the superior cerebellar artery (C).

COMPLICATIONS

Although ETV is widely accepted as a treatment for hydrocephalus, it is still a demanding approach due to several technical limitations involving depth perception, range of motion, tool dexterity, and the precarious presence of surrounding anatomical structures.[68] Intraoperative complications for ETV include neural injury (such as thalamic, forniceal, hypothalamic, and midbrain injuries), bradycardia, and hemorrhage. In an extensive review conducted by Bouras and Sgouros,

intraoperative hemorrhage was the most frequently reported ETV complication.[69] In their report, Bouras and Sgouros determined that the rate of bleeding during ETV was 3.72%, the rate of severe hemorrhage was 0.6%, and the rate of basilar rupture was 0.21%.[69] Among intraoperative bleeding events, injury to the basilar artery is considered by many to be the most dangerous complication.[2,70] When assessing a patient's anatomy for ETV surgery, in order to ensure a safe ventriculostomy, physicians should determine if there is an adequate amount of space between the basilar artery and the clivus under the floor of the third ventricle.[2] The basilar artery apex and the posterior cerebral arteries can be more readily identified by performing ETV with a pulse-waved microvascular Doppler probe and videoscope.[70] Research conducted by Wachter et al. suggests that indocyanine green angiography can also be used to identify the vessels located beneath the third ventricular floor.[71] Incorporating these kinds of imaging tools and techniques into an endoscopic procedure might help surgeons to minimize the risk of vascular injury. Bouras and Sgouros assert that hemorrhagic complications are infrequent when ETV is performed by practiced surgeons who are knowledgeable in endoscopic technique.[69] After bleeding, the second most frequently reported intraoperative event is neural injury, which had a rate of 0.24% among the cases Bouras and Sgouros examined.[69] Neural injury can be avoided by properly planning burr hole placement, avoiding side movements, and by selecting proper candidates with a significantly enlarged foramen of Monro and third ventricle.[2] In order to maximize the distance between endoscopic tools and important neuronal structures, Martinez-Moreno et al. developed a navigation protocol for ETV that involves specific imaging acquisition, trajectory planning, and continuous instrument tracking.[72] They found that implementing this protocol significantly reduced the risk of virtual stress by mechanical forces on adjacent tissue.[72]

CONCLUSION

Overall, ETV is a safe procedure associated with low rates of permanent morbidity (2.38%) and mortality (0.28%). However, there are additional steps that can be taken to ensure better patient outcomes.[69] Kulkarni et al. have developed an ETV success score (ETVSS) that can assist surgeons in estimating the probability of ETV success by factoring in each patient's age, etiology, and previous shunt experience.[58] In cases where those indications seem to contradict each other, the score sheet might be especially helpful to guide preoperative planning. The ETVSS's predictions closely align with the actual results of many infantile hydrocephalus studies published during the last 20 years.[73] Generally speaking, patients without previous shunting experience who have been diagnosed with obstructive hydrocephalus are ideal candidates for ETV as a primary treatment. Patients with hydrocephalus related to other etiologies who have had shunt placement are viable candidates for ETV as a secondary treatment. For communicating hydrocephalus cases, CPC might help increase the chance of a successful surgical outcome when it is performed in conjunction with ETV, particularly for posthemorrhagic cases or patients with a slow to moderate rate of increase in head circumference. Regardless of etiology, patients who are older than 2 months of age will likely fare better with regard to ETV surgical outcome.

REFERENCES

1. Enchev Y, Oi S. Historical trends of neuroendoscopic surgical techniques in the treatment of hydrocephalus. Neurosurgical Rev. 2008;31(3):249-62.
2. Yadav YR, Parihar V, Pande S, et al. Endoscopic third ventriculostomy. J Neurosci Rural Practice. 2012;3(2):163-73.
3. Tully HM, Dobyns WB. Infantile hydrocephalus: a review of epidemiology, classification and causes. Eur J Med Genet. 2014;57(8):359-68.
4. Greitz D. Paradigm shift in hydrocephalus research in legacy of Dandy's pioneering work: rationale for third ventriculostomy in communicating hydrocephalus. Childs Nerv Syst. 2007;23(5):487-9.
5. Oreskovic D, Klarica M. The formation of cerebrospinal fluid: nearly a hundred years of interpretations and misinterpretations. Brain Res Rev. 2010;64(2):241-62.
6. Symss NP, Oi S. Theories of cerebrospinal fluid dynamics and hydrocephalus: historical trend. J Neurosurg Pediatr. 2013;11(2):170-7.
7. Dandy WE. Where is cerebrospinal fluid absorbed? J Am Med Assoc. 1929;92(24):2012-4.
8. Greitz D, Hannerz J. A proposed model of cerebrospinal fluid circulation: observations with radionuclide cisternography. Am J Neuroradiol. 1996;17(3):431-8.
9. Greitz D, Greitz T, Hindmarsh T. A new view on the CSF-circulation with the potential for pharmacological treatment of childhood hydrocephalus. Acta Paediatrica. 1997;86(2):125-32.
10. Bulat M, Klarica M. Recent insights into a new hydrodynamics of the cerebrospinal fluid. Brain Res Rev. 2011;65(2):99-112.
11. O'Connell JE. The vascular factor in intracranial pressure and the maintenance of the cerebrospinal fluid circulation. Brain. 1943;66(3):204-28.
12. Greitz D. Radiological assessment of hydrocephalus: new theories and implications for therapy. Neurosurg Rev. 2004;27(3):145-65; discussion 66-7.
13. Greitz D. The hydrodynamic hypothesis versus the bulk flow hypothesis. Neurosurg Rev. 2004;27(4):299-300.
14. Warf BC, Campbell JW, Riddle E. Initial experience with combined endoscopic third ventriculostomy and choroid plexus cauterization for post-hemorrhagic hydrocephalus of prematurity: the importance of prepontine cistern status and the predictive value of FIESTA MRI imaging. Childs Nerv Syst. 2011;27(7):1063-71.
15. Scarff JE. Endoscopic treatment of hydrocephalus: description of a ventriculoscope and preliminary report of cases. Arch Neurol Psychiatry. 1936;35(4):853-61.
16. Lifshutz JI, Johnson WD. History of hydrocephalus and its treatments. Neurosurg Focus. 2001;11(2):E1.
17. Abbott R. History of neuroendoscopy. Neurosurg Clin N Am. 2004;15(1):1-7.
18. Patwardhan RV, Nanda A. Implanted ventricular shunts in the United States: the billion-dollar-a-year cost of hydrocephalus treatment. Neurosurgery. 2005;56(1):139-44; discussion 44-5.
19. Cinalli G. Alternatives to shunting. Childs Nerv Syst. 1999;15(11-12):718-31.
20. Zandian A, Haffner M, Johnson J, et al. Endoscopic third ventriculostomy with/without choroid plexus cauterization for hydrocephalus due to hemorrhage, infection, Dandy-Walker malformation, and neural tube defect: a meta-analysis. Childs Nerv Syst. 2014;30(4):571-8.
21. O'Brien DF, Javadpour M, Collins DR, et al. Endoscopic third ventriculostomy: an outcome analysis of primary

cases and procedures performed after ventriculoperitoneal shunt malfunction. J Neurosurg. 2005;103(5 Suppl): 393-400.

22. Cinalli G, Sainte-Rose C, Chumas P, et al. Failure of third ventriculostomy in the treatment of aqueductal stenosis in children. J Neurosurg. 1999;90(3):448-54.

23. Mugamba J, Stagno V. Indication for endoscopic third ventriculostomy. World Neurosurg. 2013;79(2 Suppl):S20 e19-23.

24. Tisell M, Almström O, Stephensen H, et al. How effective is endoscopic third ventriculostomy in treating adult hydrocephalus caused by primary aqueductal stenosis? Neurosurgery. 2000;46(1):104-11.

25. El Beltagy MA, Kamal HM, Taha H, et al. Endoscopic third ventriculostomy before tumor surgery in children with posterior fossa tumors, CCHE experience. Childs Nerv Syst.. 2010;26(12):1699-704.

26. Ruggiero C, Cinalli G, Spennato P, et al. Endoscopic third ventriculostomy in the treatment of hydrocephalus in posterior fossa tumors in children. Childs Nerv Syst. 2004;20(11-12):828-33.

27. Sainte-Rose C, Cinalli G, Roux FE, et al. Management of hydrocephalus in pediatric patients with posterior fossa tumors: the role of endoscopic third ventriculostomy. J Neurosurg. 2001;95(5):791-7.

28. O'Brien DF, Hayhurst C, Pizer B, et al. Outcomes in patients undergoing single-trajectory endoscopic third ventriculostomy and endoscopic biopsy for midline tumors presenting with obstructive hydrocephalus. J Neurosurg. 2006;105(3 Suppl):219-26.

29. Roopesh Kumar SV, Mohanty A, Santosh V, et al. Endoscopic options in management of posterior third ventricular tumors. Childs Nerv Syst. 2007;23(10):1135-45.

30. du Plessis AJ. The role of systemic hemodynamic disturbances in prematurity-related brain injury. J Child Neurol. 2009;24(9):1127-40.

31. Chamiraju P, Bhatia S, Sandberg DI, et al. Endoscopic third ventriculostomy and choroid plexus cauterization in posthemorrhagic hydrocephalus of prematurity. J Neurosurg Pediatr. 2014;13(4):433-9.

32. Siomin V, Cinalli G, Grotenhuis A, et al. Endoscopic third ventriculostomy in patients with cerebrospinal fluid infection and/or hemorrhage. J Neurosurg. 2002;97(3):519-24.

33. Oertel JM, Mondorf Y, Baldauf J, et al. Endoscopic third ventriculostomy for obstructive hydrocephalus due to intracranial hemorrhage with intraventricular extension. J Neurosurg. 2009;111(6):1119-26.

34. Stone SS, Warf BC. Combined endoscopic third ventriculostomy and choroid plexus cauterization as primary treatment for infant hydrocephalus: a prospective North American series. J Neurosurg Pediatr. 2014;14(5):439-46.

35. Fukuhara T, Vorster SJ, Luciano MG. Risk factors for failure of endoscopic third ventriculostomy for obstructive hydrocephalus. Neurosurgery. 2000;46(5):1100-9; discussion 9-11.

36. Schwartz TH, Yoon SS, Cutruzzola FW, et al. Third ventriculostomy: post-operative ventricular size and outcome. Minim Invasive Neurosurg. 1996;39(4):122-9.

37. Warf BC. Hydrocephalus in Uganda: the predominance of infectious origin and primary management with endoscopic third ventriculostomy. J Neurosurg. 2005;102(1 Suppl):1-15.

38. Warf BC, Kulkarni AV. Intraoperative assessment of cerebral aqueduct patency and cisternal scarring: impact on success of endoscopic third ventriculostomy in 403 African children. J Neurosurg Pediatr. 2010;5(2):204-9.

39. Sufianov AA, Sufianova GZ, Iakimov IA. Endoscopic third ventriculostomy in patients younger than 2 years: outcome analysis of 41 hydrocephalus cases. J Neurosurg Pediatr. 2010;5(4):392-401.

40. Chadduck W, Adametz J. Incidence of seizures in patients with myelomeningocele: a multifactorial analysis. Surg Neurol. 1988;30(4):281-5.

41. Reddy GK, Bollam P, Caldito G. Ventriculoperitoneal shunt surgery and the risk of shunt infection in patients with hydrocephalus: long-term single institution experience. World Neurosurg. 2012;78(1-2):155-63.

42. Walters BC, Hoffman HJ, Hendrick EB, et al. Cerebrospinal fluid shunt infection. Influences on initial management and subsequent outcome. J Neurosurg. 1984;60(5):1014-21.

43. McGirt MJ, Zaas A, Fuchs HE, et al. Risk factors for pediatric ventriculoperitoneal shunt infection and predictors of infectious pathogens. Clin Infect Dis. 2003;36(7):858-62.

44. Casey AT, Kimmings EJ, Kleinlugtebeld AD, et al. The long-term outlook for hydrocephalus in childhood. A ten-year cohort study of 155 patients. Pediatric Neurosurg. 1997;27(2):63-70.

45. Spennato P, Ruggiero C, Aliberti F, et al. Third ventriculostomy in shunt malfunction. World Neurosurg. 2013;79(2 Suppl):S22.e21-6.

46. Baskin JJ, Manwaring KH, Rekate HL. Ventricular shunt removal: the ultimate treatment of the slit ventricle syndrome. J Neurosurg. 1998;88(3):478-84.

47. Jones RF, Stening WA, Kwok BC, et al. Third ventriculostomy for shunt infections in children. Neurosurgery. 1993;32(5):855-9; discussion 60.

48. Cinalli G, Salazar C, Mallucci C, et al. The role of endoscopic third ventriculostomy in the management of shunt malfunction. Neurosurgery. 1998;43(6):1323-7; discussion 7-9.

49. Scarrow AM, Levy EI, Pascucci L, et al. Outcome analysis of endoscopic III ventriculostomy. Childs Nerv Syst.. 2000;16(7):442-4; discussion 5.

50. Teo C, Jones R. Management of hydrocephalus by endoscopic third ventriculostomy in patients with myelomeningocele. Pediatric Neurosurg. 1996;25(2):57-63.

51. Rivero-Garvia M, Marquez-Rivas J, Rueda Torres AB, et al. Cranial growth restriction, a fundamental measure for success of the endoscopy in children under 1 month of age. Is it possible to improve the outcome? J Pediatr Surg. 2013;48(7):1628-32.

52. Baldauf J, Oertel J, Gaab MR, et al. Endoscopic third ventriculostomy in children younger than 2 years of age. Childs Nerv Syst. 2007;23(6):623-6.

53. Faggin R, Bernardo A, Stieg P, et al. Hydrocephalus in infants less than six months of age: effectiveness of endoscopic third ventriculostomy. Eur J Pediatr Surg. 2009;19(4):216-9.

54. Ogiwara H, Dipatri AJ Jr, Alden TD, et al. Endoscopic third ventriculostomy for obstructive hydrocephalus in children younger than 6 months of age. Childs Nerv Syst. 2010;26(3):343-7.

55. Gallo P, Szathmari A, De Biasi S, et al. Endoscopic third ventriculostomy in obstructive infantile hydrocephalus: remarks about the so-called 'unsuccessful cases'. Pediatr Neurosurg. 2010;46(6):435-41.

56. Lewis AI, Keiper GL Jr, Crone KR. Endoscopic treatment of loculated hydrocephalus. J Neurosurg. 1995;82(5):780-5.

57. El-Ghandour NM. Endoscopic cyst fenestration in the treatment of uniloculated hydrocephalus in children. J Neurosurg Pediatr. 2013;11(4):402-9.

58. Kulkarni AV, Drake JM, Mallucci CL, et al. Endoscopic third ventriculostomy in the treatment of childhood hydrocephalus. J Pediatr. 2009;155(2):254-9.e1.

59. Warf BC. Comparison of endoscopic third ventriculostomy alone and combined with choroid plexus cauterization in infants younger than 1 year of age: a prospective study in 550 African children. J Neurosurg. 2005;103(6 Suppl): 475-81.

60. Dandy WE. Extirpation of the choroid plexus of the lateral ventricles in communicating hydrocephalus. Ann Surg. 1918;68(6):569-79.

61. Putnam TJ. Treatment of hydrocephalus by endoscopic coagulation of the choroid plexus: description of a new instrument and preliminary report of results. N Eng J Med. 1934;210(26):1373-6.

62. Scarff JE. The treatment of nonobstructive (communicating) hydrocephalus by endoscopic cauterization of the choroid plexuses. J Neurosurg. 1970;33(1):1-18.

63. Pople IK, Ettles D. The role of endoscopic choroid plexus coagulation in the management of hydrocephalus. Neurosurgery. 1995;36(4):698-701; discussion 701-2.

64. Morota N, Fujiyama Y. Endoscopic coagulation of choroid plexus as treatment for hydrocephalus: indication and surgical technique. Childs Nerv Syst. 2004;20(11-12): 816-20.

65. Warf BC, Campbell JW. Combined endoscopic third ventriculostomy and choroid plexus cauterization as primary treatment of hydrocephalus for infants with myelomeningocele: long-term results of a prospective intent-to-treat study in 115 East African infants. J Neurosurg Pediatr. 2008;2(5):310-6.

66. Turner L. The structure of arachnoid granulations with observations on their physiological and pathological significance. Ann R Coll Surg Engl. 1961;29:237-64.

67. Oi S, Di Rocco C. Proposal of "evolution theory in cerebrospinal fluid dynamics" and minor pathway hydrocephalus in developing immature brain. Childs Nerv Syst. 2006;22(7):662-9.

68. Breimer GE, Bodani V, Looi T, et al. Design and evaluation of a new synthetic brain simulator for endoscopic third ventriculostomy. J Neurosurg Pediatr. 2015;15(1):82-8.

69. Bouras T, Sgouros S. Complications of endoscopic third ventriculostomy. J Neurosurg Pediatr. 2011;7(6):643-9.

70. Eguchi S, Aihara Y, Tsuzuki S, et al. A modified method to enhance the safety of endoscopic third ventriculostomy (ETV)—transendoscopic pulse-waved microvascular Doppler-assisted ETV, technical note. Childs Nerv Syst. 2014;30(3):515-9.

71. Wachter D, Behm T, von Eckardstein K, et al. Indocyanine green angiography in endoscopic third ventriculostomy. Neurosurgery. 2013;73(1 Suppl Operative):ons67-72; ons72-3.

72. Martinez-Moreno M, Widhalm G, Mert A, et al. A novel protocol of continuous navigation guidance for endoscopic third ventriculostomy. Neurosurgery. 2014;10(Suppl 4):514-23; discussion 23-4.

73. Kulkarni AV, Riva-Cambrin J, Browd SR. Use of the ETV Success Score to explain the variation in reported endoscopic third ventriculostomy success rates among published case series of childhood hydrocephalus. J Neurosurg Pediatr. 2011;7(2):143-6.

CHAPTER 6

Endoscopic Treatment of Symptomatic Midline Cavum Septum Pellucidum Cysts

David F Jimenez, David N Garza

INTRODUCTION

The septum pellucidum is a solid or membranous bridge located between the corpus callosum and the fornix that relays visceral information through the hypothalamic autonomic system to the hippocampus, amygdala, habenula, and brainstem reticular formation; it is involved in consciousness, sleep, and emotional responses to our environment.[1,2] The septum pellucidum is composed of two individual septal laminae that are often described as leaflets. During fetal development, these leaflets are separated by a sagittally oriented, fluid-filled cavity called the cavum septum pellucidum (CSP)[3] (Figs. 1 and 2). As the fetus matures, the leaflets fuse together in a caudal to cranial orientation and the CSP closes[4] (Fig. 3).

Although this closure is considered a standard phase of development, the cavity's persistence after birth is a relatively normal anatomical variation that has been observed in 85% of 1-month-old infants and up to 20% of adults (Fig. 4). The presence of some lingering remnant of the cavum in adults is not considered by many authors to be extraordinary, but the reported incidence of this occurrence within the literature actually varies quite dramatically due to the absence of a standard anatomical definition for CSP and differing detection methodologies.[5,6] The incidence cited by Souweidane et al., for example, ranged from 4% to 74% (Figs. 5A and B).

While it is usually a benign structure, the CSP might warrant surgical intervention if it enlarges and becomes symptomatic. When that happens, the CSP will often

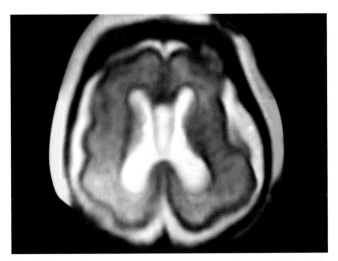

Fig. 1: Magnetic resonance imaging coronal image of 26-week-old fetus showing the widely, manually separated leaflets of the septum pellucidum.

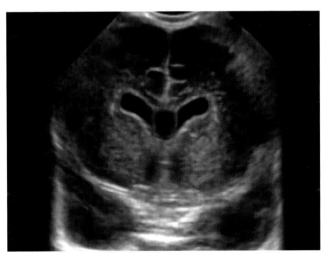

Fig. 2: Magnetic resonance imaging axial image of 33-week-old fetus showing progressive approximation of the septal leaflets.

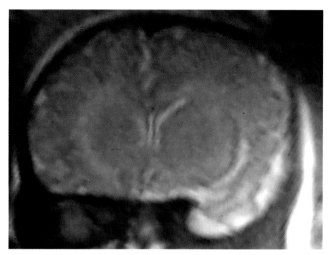

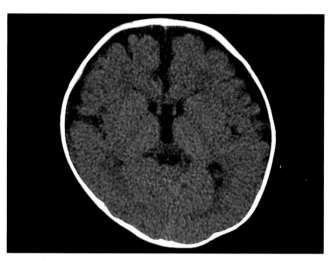

Fig. 3: Magnetic resonance imaging coronal image of a full term infant showing almost complete fusion of septal leaflets.

Fig. 4: Normal persistence of an asymptomatic cavum septum pellucidum in a 3-year-old child. Such cavities do not require any type of surgical intervention.

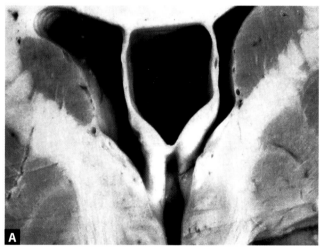

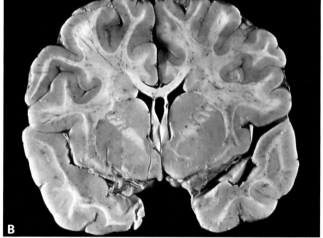

Figs. 5A and B: (A) Photograph of pathologic brain section of a 68-year-old male with an incidental cavum septum pellucidum at autopsy. (B) Coronal brain section of a young adult with asymptomatic cavum.
Courtesy: James Henry MD.

be described as a cyst, a congenital cerebral cyst of the cavum, or a dilated or widened cavum.[6,7] If left untreated, the enlarged CSP (or cyst) can cause significant neurological dysfunction due to its obstruction of the intraventricular foramina, distortion of the vascular structures of the deep venous system, and compression of the hypothalamoseptal triangle.[8] At this time, there is not a commonly accepted standard that surgeons can apply to clearly distinguish a large CSP from a cyst of the septum pellucidum. However, Sarwar and other authors have suggested that a septum pellucidum cyst can be more precisely defined as

a fluid-filled structure between the lateral ventricles with walls that exhibit lateral bowing and extend 10 mm apart or greater[1,9] (Fig. 6). Unlike those of a cyst, the walls of cavi septi pellucidi are often described as being parallel to each other. Symptoms are not expected to manifest if the cyst walls are 5 mm apart or less.[1]

The persistence of the CSP into later stages of development is uncommon. Its progression into a symptomatic, dilated cyst is rarer still. Wang et al. reported that among 54,000 patients who underwent cranial computed tomography (CT) and magnetic resonance imaging (MRI), only

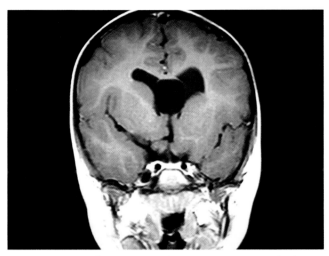

Fig. 6: CT scan of a 19-year-old male presenting with chronic and severe headaches. It depicts an enlarged CSP. (CT: Computed tomography; CSP: Cavum septum pellucidum).

22 had a dilated cyst of the CSP (an incidence of 0.04%).[7] Communicating cysts of the septum pellucidum do not usually bear any clinical significance because they are unlikely to reach an extraordinary size; noncommunicating cysts, however, can enlarge and block the foramina of Monro, which could lead to the buildup of cerebrospinal fluid (CSF) and the development of hydrocephalus.[2,10] Recognition of this distinction has led some authors to classify cysts of the septum pellucidum as either (1) incidental, asymptomatic, communicating cysts or (2) pathological, symptomatic, noncommunicating cysts with increased intracystic pressure.[6,10] The cysts might further be described as either "simple" or "complex" depending on whether or not they are associated with neurological lesions.[6]

The first published observations of dilated septum pellucidum cavities were likely reported by Jacobus Sylvius in the 15th century.[11,12] Meyer is often credited for being the first person to describe the pneumoencephalographic appearance of the CSP in 1930; however, Pendergrass and Hodes as well as Love and Lowman also conducted studies and made similar observations around the same time.[12,13] Surgical intervention for cysts of the septum pellucidum can be traced back to Dandy who, in 1931, reported two cases that he treated by creating communication between the cyst and the lateral ventricle through the corpus callosum anterior to the Rolandic vein.[12] Around 1934, Van Wagen and Aird operated on a

cyst of the septum pellucidum by approaching the lateral ventricle transcortically through the frontal lobe; the cyst was perforated and communication was restored but, 2 months later, symptoms recurred and a complete remission did not follow until after they performed a series of ventricular punctures.[12] They went on to report six more cases of noncommunicating cavity of the septum, but all were discovered incidentally at necropsy.[12]

Van Wagen and Aird along with some of their contemporaries suggested that encephalography and ventriculography might be responsible for rupturing cysts of the septum pellucidum during imaging studies.[12,13] After the emergence of CT and MRI, cysts of the septum pellucidum became much easier to diagnose, but the condition was still rarely reported.[14] Between 1931 and 2012, within English language literature, there were only 31 documented cases of symptomatic CSP cysts in children under the age of 18 that were also confirmed with imaging studies.[15]

TREATMENT

Up until 1999, cysts of the septum pellucidum were traditionally treated using open surgical procedures, such as craniotomy and cyst fenestration (via a transcallosal or transcortical approach), conventional shunting (ventriculoperitoneal or cystoperitoneal), and stereotactic fenestration.[15] However, each of these techniques has certain risks and limitations associated with them. It has been suggested by some authors that because the caves of the septum pellucidum can potentially reform after direct fenestration and possibly cause a recurrence of symptoms, shunting might be the simplest and most reliable form of treatment.[13,16] Others argue that shunting might ultimately prove to be an ineffective long-term solution because CSP has previously been cited as a possible cause of shunt malfunction.[17] Additionally, one must take into consideration the morbidity associated with shunting: the potential for venous hemorrhage, infarction, and blind puncture of the cyst wall.[18] Stereotactic procedures are problematic because visual inspection of the foramen of Monro is not possible; if there are any lingering adhesions between the cyst and the lateral ventricle, they may contribute to the recurrence of hydrocephalus after the apparently successful drainage of the cyst.[18]

In 1995, Jackowski et al. described a new approach to septum pellucidotomy that used a flexible neuroendoscope and a laser to fenestrate a midline cyst in an adult male.[15,19] This trailblazing event was viewed with some skepticism a few years later when Lancon et al. called into question Jackowski's diagnosis in their 1999 publication of the first endoscopic approach used to treat a CSP cyst in a child.[20] Since that time, 16 years ago, endoscopy has become a much more commonplace technique. Between 1999 and 2012, all 15 reported cases of radiologically-confirmed, symptomatic CSP cyst in children were treated using endoscopic methods; all of them fully recovered or improved following treatment.[15] Endoscopy is now, quite clearly, the preferred surgical option for the treatment of cysts of the septum pellucidum.

Endoscopic fenestration of the CSP is an ideal approach to surgical intervention because it creates communication between the cyst and the ventricular system while avoiding the complications of shunting and open craniotomies.[18] The two main advantages of endoscope-assisted surgery compared to microsurgical techniques are: (1) a reduction of superficial brain retraction with less iatrogenic trauma to neighboring structures and (2) the simultaneous depiction of anatomical details and changes that are not visible with a microscope under the same conditions.[21] Endoscopy offers shorter operations times (roughly 1 hour in duration) that are less invasive for the patient than traditional techniques.[22] Having enhanced, direct visualization provides surgeons with the ability to observe the positional relation of the veins in the wall of the CSP and inspect the interventricular foramina of Monro for potential adhesions, evidence of fibrosis, or intermittent obstruction by flaccid cyst walls.[13,22] Endoscopic technique also enables the surgeon to perform biopsies of the cyst walls, which can be helpful for pathological studies.[22]

Complications following endoscopy are rare. Of the 15 reported cases referenced earlier, there was only one instance of mild bleeding during surgery.[15,23] The main difficulty encountered by surgeons during the endoscopic fenestration of CSP cysts was the loss of a precise target to establish communication between the cyst and the ventricles.[15] There are, however, tools that can compensate for that disadvantage, such as neuronavigation systems and ultrasound.[24,25] These devices and their accompanying techniques provide even more accuracy and guidance during surgery. Neuronavigation-assisted endoscopy, in particular, can help surgeons determine the best operative trajectory and locate the ventricular horn, which is often very small in these patients because of the bowing cyst walls.[15] Chiu et al. have reported positive outcomes while performing navigator-assisted endoscopic fenestration of one side of a cystic wall. They have claimed it to be simple, safe, and effective, providing dramatic symptomatic relief with limited to no complications and recurrence.[24]

Although opening only one wall of the cyst has yielded good results for some authors, Borha et al. indicate that, ideally, both cyst walls should be opened once the surgeon is inside the ventricle.[15,24,26,27] One specific instance in which neuronavigation might be able to assist surgeons with enhanced visualization is after the initial perforation of the cyst wall; the subsequent perforation of the contralateral wall is often more difficult to achieve due to the proximity of contralateral neural structures and the lack of tension in the wall after the cyst has been opened.[15] Neuronavigation could facilitate the second perforation, but that application is the subject of debate. Some authors question whether or not neuronavigation can actually make a substantial difference under these circumstances because its accuracy will necessarily be affected by any shift that occurs in the brain or cyst wall.[18] I have found in my experience treating 23 symptomatic CSP that fenestration of a single ipsilateral leaflet is sufficient in obtaining successful long-lasting results. Attempting to fenestrate the contralateral leaflet is challenging and risky.

Visualization is important because one of the goals surgeons have when treating a CSP cyst is finding a safe, avascular region in which they can perform a septostomy. However, many authors have debated precisely where that region is located. Besides that, each patient must also be assessed individually so that their unique anatomical properties (dimensions of septum pellucidum, location of abnormality, size, and orientation of contralateral ventricle) are taken into consideration before a location is finally chosen.[28]

Because the degree of vascularity is so relevant to determining where the best place to perform the septostomy is, Roth et al. conducted a study examining the arrangement of septal veins. They ultimately concluded that their distribution was, contrary to popular belief, asymmetric in most cases and suggested that surgeons should consider performing the septostomy near the anterior area of the middle septal region at the level of the foramen of Monro, mid-height between the corpus callosum, and the fornix.[28] Many surgeons undertake an anterior approach to cyst fenestration, but cannulation of the anterior horn can be difficult in symptomatic cases that are not accompanied by hydrocephalus.[22] Miki et al.

used an anterior approach through a right frontal burr hole in their series of CSP cases but, in order to create working spaces that aided maneuverability, they inflated collapsed cyst cavities with Ringer's lactate solution during irrigation and used flexible fiberscopes.[22] They found this approach to be safe and easy to perform, but considered it to be a feasible only in symptomatic CSP cases.[22] I agree with them that there is great variability in the position of septal veins and as such, I decide where to place the ostomy after full visualization of the septum and selecting an avascular area.

Even when the cannulation is successfully performed in the anterior horn, some authors report that fenestration of the CSP cyst is precarious due to the acute angle; there is a chance the surgeon might injure the fornix, thalamus, internal capsule, caudate nucleus, and septal and thalamostriate veins.[22] Lancon et al. report that cannulation of the lateral ventricle before cyst fenestration prevents inadvertent injury to the aforementioned structures.[20] Likewise, Gangemi et al. have suggested that surgeons use a posterior approach through a right occipital burr hole in order to easily cannulate the occipital horn and avoid damaging the neural and vascular structures surrounding the foramen of Monro.[27] My approach is to place the entry burr hole frontally but significantly more lateral that the standard Kocher's point, as will be described later in the chapter.

When implementing an endoscopic surgical approach to the third ventricle, special considerations must be made when a patient has a CSP. The cavum's presence results in the lateral displacement of the septal leaflets and an inferior, lateral shift of the forniceal columns, which effects two major anatomical changes: (1) a reduction in the width of the lateral ventricle that encumbers the cannulation of the lateral ventricle and (2) the diminishment or occlusion of the foramen of Monro by the forniceal column.[4] Because these obstacles preclude a safe transforaminal approach into the third ventricle, Souweidane et al. suggest that surgeons undertake a transcavum interforniceal route instead with the rostral lamina and anterior commissure acting as important anatomical landmarks.[4]

CLINICAL PRESENTATION

Cysts of the septum pellucidum have been associated with a wide range of symptoms and neuropsychiatric disorders, including acute hydrocephalus, loss of consciousness, autonomic dysfunctions, seizures, psychiatric problems, visual/behavioral/sensorimotor disturbances, and intermittent headaches.[7,23] Patients who retain an enlarged CSP present with similar symptoms. In a study conducted by Akiyama et al., patients with a CSP who were surveyed indicated headache as their chief complaint, followed by nausea and/or vomiting, epileptic attacks, dizziness, and emotional instability.[29] Epileptic seizures have been described in 31% to 55% of CSP cases and psychosis, dementia, and personality changes have been described in about 15% of CSP cases; other symptoms, like giddiness, intracranial pressure, and hemiparesis have also been recorded.[1] In their 2007 study, Flashman et al. determined that the presence of a CSP was not strictly associated with schizophrenia; however, patients with schizophrenia who also had an abnormally large CSP did appear to exhibit greater symptom severity and cognitive defects in areas such as intellectual functioning and verbal learning and memory.[30] However a cause and effect relationship has not been established.

The symptom presentation for this patient population is so diverse because of the various pathological outcomes that can be created by mass effect or the disturbance of the emotional and behavioral functions of the limbic system.[5] There are primarily three physiopathological mechanisms that describe how and why CSP cyst symptoms manifest. The first mechanism is an increase in intracranial pressure as a result of a cyst obstructing the intraventricular foramina through the ball valve phenomenon.[13,22] The second is the compression of the hypothalamoseptal triangle, including the specific septal nuclei, periseptal nuclei, and associated projection pathways related to neuropsychiatric symptoms and the compression of optic chiasm and pathways.[13,15] The final mechanism is chronic deep venous impairment; the stretching and displacement of internal cerebral and subependymal veins has been linked to progressive focal deficits.[13-15,22]

For many physicians, the main diagnostic challenge when confronted with this wide range of presentations is clearly establishing a correlation between the patient's symptoms and the cyst. The physician must determine if the cyst is an isolated, symptomatic lesion, a symptomatic cyst coincident with another symptomatic disease, or an incidental finding in a patient with another disease process.[13] A patient's medical history as well as their clinical presentation, radiological demonstrations, and intracranial pressure must all be evaluated carefully before a treatment can be selected.[23] In my practice the main and primary reason for recommending surgery to a patient

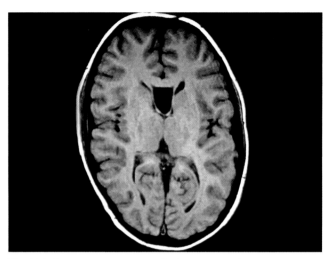

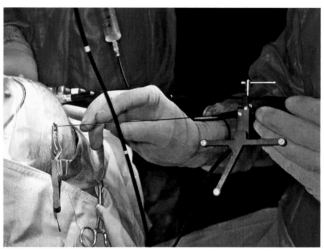

Fig. 7: It is not uncommon to find symptomatic cavum septum pellucidum with very small frontal horns and no hydrocephalus. In those cases the use of neuronavigation is extremely important. Once the ventricle is accessed, it can be gently and slowly inflated with lactated ringers.

Fig. 8: Fiberscope coupled with neuronavigation used to cannulate frontal horn of patient in Figure 7.

is the presence of chronic, unremittent headaches, particularly if they are made worse with tussive maneuvers (coughing, bending over, etc.).

In their study of CSP cysts, Miki et al. concluded that headache due to increased intracranial pressure or clinical symptoms attributed to the compression of the limbic system, basal ganglia, optic chiasm, and deep veins, coupled with proof of a noncommunicating, expanding CSP via CT cisternography constituted reasonable evidence to establish a diagnosis of symptomatic CSP.[22] However, it should be noted that not all patients with headache symptoms or evidence of increased intracranial pressure present with evidence of hydrocephalus.[15] Headache in patients without hydrocephalus could be the result of the cyst's intermittent obstruction of the interventricular foramina, for example.[23] In a study conducted by Borha et al., only 32.3% of children with radiologically confirmed, symptomatic CSP cysts presented with hydrocephalus.[15]

Wester et al. have proposed that the relationship between hydrocephalus and CSP cysts could be more complex than many have suspected. They reported two cases of CSP cysts and concomitant hydrocephalus that were not improved following stereotactic cystoventricular shunt placement, which lead them to believe that the growth of the cavum might actually be the result, rather than the cause, of hydrocephalus.[15,31] Because physicians are still trying to understand the relationship between hydrocephalus symptoms and the pathology of CSP cysts,

the absence of clinical signs of hydrocephalus in a patient with behavioral, autonomic, or sensorimotor symptoms should not strictly be considered a contraindication for surgical decompression.[13]

As previously stated, my personal experience having treated patients with symptomatic CSP cysts is that headache is the primary indication for treatment. One hundred percent of patients presented with headaches while they also presented with other symptoms. Endoscopic fenestration has resulted in resolution of the headaches (without recurrence) in 100% of the patients. My practice is primarily to fenestrate the ipsilateral (largest frontal horn if asymmetric) septal leaf. Whenever possible, the contralateral leaf is fenestrated but is not necessary.

TECHNIQUE

After induction of the patient under general anesthesia, the patient is placed supine with the head on a horseshoe head holder in a neutral position in both the sagittal and coronal planes. If available, image guidance neuronavigational assistance may be used but is not necessary unless dealing with extremely small ventricles (Figs. 7 and 8). A preoperative MRI can be used for proper burr hole localization using all three planes: (1) sagittal, (2) coronal, and (3) axial. Unlike most frontal horn endoscopic surgery that utilizes a Kocher's point of entrance, endoscopic access for CSP utilizes a burr hole that is more laterally

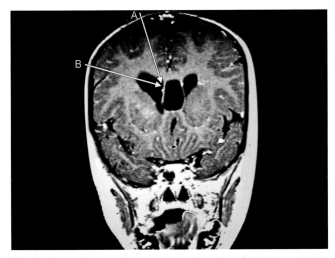

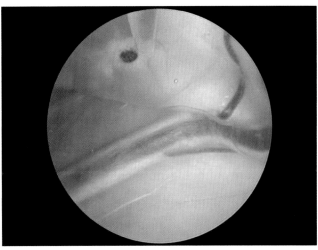

Fig. 9: Coronal magnetic resonance imaging showing access to the frontal horn via a standard approach (A) and a more laterally placed approach (B). The former gives the surgeon a suboptimal angle and increases risk of fornix and the other neural injury. The latter (B) is the best option as it provides the surgeon with a direct, en-face view of the septum, fornix, and septal veins.

Fig. 10: A small opening has been created on the leaf of the septum pellucidum with a 350 micron YAG laser fiber. This is done in a circumferential fashion until the outline of the full ostomy is obtained.

located (between 6 cm and 8 cm from midline) (Fig. 9). The goal is to access the frontal horn as to have direct visualization of the septum (perpendicular approach). I agree with Miki et al.[22] that critical structures can be damaged with a traditional Kocher's point approach due to the parallel aspect of this approach.

The ventricle should be first cannulated with a ventricular catheter to ascertain proper trajectory and access to the ventricle. Opening pressure should be performed with a manometer and CSF sample obtained. Following removal of the ventricular catheter, a 14 French peel-away catheter (or the cannula of the endoscopic system in use) is introduced using the same trajectory and depth. The obturator is removed and a zero degree endoscope is introduced. Typically the ventricles are small as is the working space and the septal leaf will be in direct view. Irrigation is now used to determine the location of the leaf which will mobilize easily back and forth with direct and intermittent irrigation. If the scope is facing the corpus callosum or other solid neural structure, it will not sway or move with direct intermittent irrigation. Inspection of the septal leaf will show location of the septal veins. Fenestration should be done between these veins at their greatest area of separation. Although my first choice for fenestration is a laser, it can be done with a Bugby wire, monopolar or direct puncture of the wall. However, direct puncture only places the patient at risk for closure as

the free floating septal leaves can come in contact with each other and fuse. A successful technique to create the ostomy includes setting the power source (laser, monopolar, etc.) at low wattage and directly contacting the leaflet, creating a full thickness small hole (Fig. 10). The same maneuver is done in an area next to it and moving in a circumferential fashion. This creates the outline of the osteotomy (Fig. 11). However, commonly, cauterized pieces of septal leaf remain on the edges of the ostomy. A pair of grasping or biopsy forceps are used to remove the debris and fully open the ostomy (Fig. 12). Finally, the laser is used to fully cauterize the ostomy edges to obtain a fully patent opening (Fig. 13).

After the ostomy is made, the field is fully irrigated with lactated ringers solution and the endoscope is advanced into the CSP and its contents visualized. At conclusion, all the instrumentation is removed. If inadvertent bleeding has occurred from injuring a small vein, an external ventricular drain may be left in place for 24–36 hours to drain the blood and clear the CSF. Fortunately, this is not a common occurrence. The galea is closed with absorbable sutures and the scalp with staples or nylon nonabsorbable suture. The patient is closely observed overnight and in almost all cases can be discharged from the hospital on the first postoperative day. I use grasping forceps to remove septal leaf tissue and cauterize the fenestration edges to prevent reclosure. The endoscope and cannulas

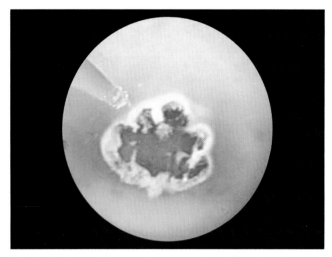

Fig. 11: Endoscopic image shows complete delineation of ostomy with the laser in circumferential fashion.

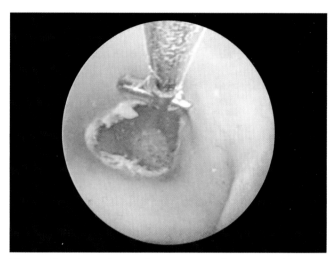

Fig. 12: Grasping or biopsy forceps are used to remove fulgirized debris on the edges of the ostomy as shown on this endoscopic view.

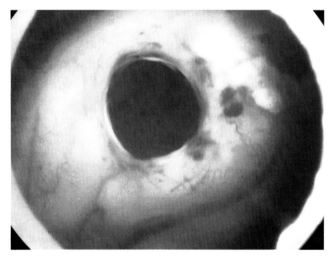

Fig. 13: Endoscopic view of an ostomy of the septal leaflet. It was performed with a YAG laser. After removing the center tissue, the edges are carefully cauterized in a circumferential fashion in order to obtain a wide opening that will not reocclude.

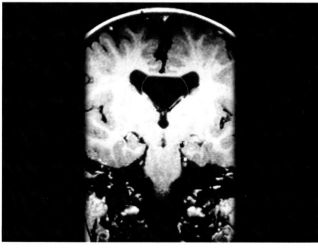

Fig. 14: Magnetic resonance imaging (MRI), coronal T1 of case 1 patient at level of foramen of Monro, shows a dilated cavum septum pellucidum (CSP) with expanded, showed out leaflets and elevation and flattening of the body of the corpus callosum.

are removed and a burr hole cover is used followed by scalp closure. Most surgeries can be done within an hour.

CLINICAL CASES

Case 1

Twenty-five-year-old female who presented with 10 years history of progressively worse bifrontal headaches. Cephalgia was made worse with bending forward and

sudden movements to the sides. Neurological examination was negative. Work up with MRI (Figs. 14 and 15) demonstrated an enlarged cyst of the septum pellucidum. A septum pellucidomy led to full resolution of symptoms immediately following surgery.

Case 2

Eighteen-year-old male presented with chronic headaches of 4 years duration. Pain became progressively more severe and patient also complained of pressure in

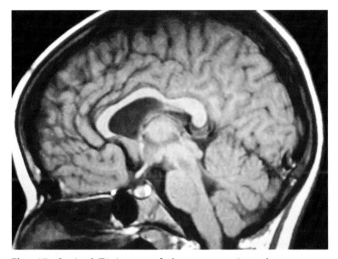

Fig. 15: Sagittal T1 image of the same patient demonstrates significant elevation of the body of the corpus callosum at the level of the cyst, indicating that the cyst was under focal pressure.

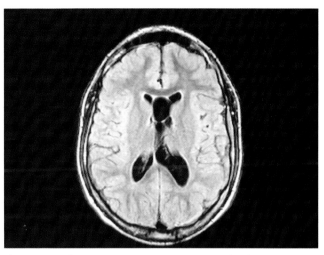

Fig. 16: Axial magnetic resonance imaging (MRI) preoperative demonstrates an expanded cavum septum pellucidum (CSP) without enlargement of the frontal horns. Note that the left frontal horn is slightly larger than the right, thus the left-sided approach.

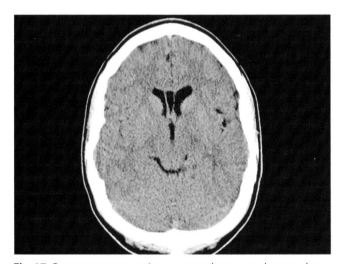

Fig. 17: One year postoperative computed tomography scan shows that the leafs of the septum are straight and a small persistent ostomy is seen on the left leaf. Patient was asymptomatic.

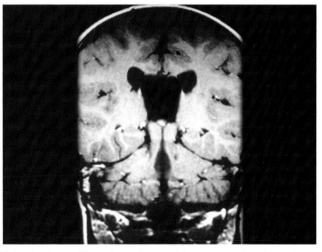

Fig. 18: Coronal T1-weighted magnetic resonance imaging shows large midline cavi.

his head. Diagnostic MRI found an expanded CSP with minor oblation of occipital horns but not of the frontal horns (Fig. 16). He underwent a left sided septum pellucidomy and a year later showed complete symptom resolution as well as a deflated CSP (Fig. 17).

Case 3

Fourteen-year-old female presented with severe global headaches for past 2 years prior. Magnetic resonance

imaging showed a combination of CSP and cavum vergae (Figs. 18 and 19). An endoscopic fenestration was done posteriorly leading to full symptom resolution at 3 years follow-up (Fig. 20).

Case 4

Twenty-year-old female presented with chronic headaches and progressive blurring of vision. Preoperative MRI showed a widely enlarged cavum vergae (Fig. 21).

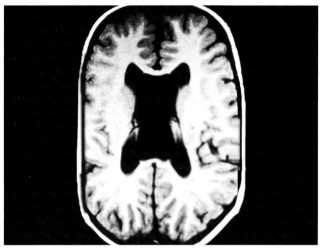

Fig. 19: Axial T1 magnetic resonance imaging (MRI) shows a cavum septum pellucidum (CSP) that extended from genu of corpus callosum (a combination of pellucidum and vergae cavi).

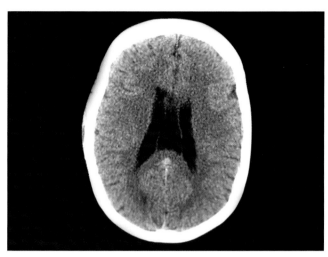

Fig. 20: Axial computed tomography scan 3 years postoperative shows straightening of the septal leafs and complete symptom resolution clinically.

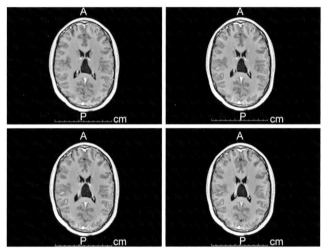

Fig. 21: Axial T1 magnetic resonance imaging shows an enlarged cavum vergae.

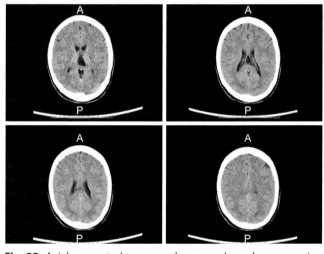

Fig. 22: Axial computed tomography scans show decompression of cavum vergae.

She underwent an endoscopic cyst fenestration and became asymptomatic. A CT scan a year later showed a decompressed cavum vergae (Fig. 22).

CONCLUSION

Cysts of the septum pellucidum are rare but treatable. An endoscopic approach to surgery provides better visibility and an overall experience that is less invasive for the patient. The procedure has a high rate of success and avoids risks related to shunting and open craniotomy.

Complications are rare, but many authors believe that neuronavigation systems and ultrasound can help surgeons compensate for any difficulties they might encounter with better operative planning and visualization.

Many surgeons prefer an anterior approach to cyst fenestration, but cannulation of the anterior horn can be difficult to accomplish in cases that are not accompanied by hydrocephalus. Under those circumstances, several authors have suggested that surgeons take a posterior approach and cannulate the occipital horn in order to avoid damaging any neural and vascular structures surrounding the foramina of Monro.

REFERENCES

1. Sarwar M. The septum pellucidum: normal and abnormal. AJNR Am J Neuroradiol. 1989;10(5):989-1005.

2. Amin B. Symptomatic cyst of the septum pellucidum. Childs Nerv Syst. 1986;2(6):320-2.

3. Tubbs RS, Krishnamurthy S, Verma K, et al. Cavum velum interpositum, cavum septum pellucidum, and cavum vergae: a review. Childs Nerv Syst. 2011;27(11):1927-30.

4. Souweidane MM, Hoffman CE, Schwartz TH. Transcavum interforniceal endoscopic surgery of the third ventricle. J Neurosurg Pediat. 2008;2(4):231-6.

5. Silbert PL, Gubbay SS, Vaughan RJ. Cavum septum pellucidum and obstructive hydrocephalus. J Neurol Neurosurg Psychiat. 1993;56(7):820-2.

6. Shaw CM, Alvord EC Jr. Cava septi pellucidi et vergae: their normal and pathological states. Brain. 1969;92(1):213-23.

7. Wang KC, Fuh JL, Lirng JF, et al. Headache profiles in patients with a dilatated cyst of the cavum septi pellucidi. Cephalalgia. 2004;24(10):867-74.

8. Fratzoglou M, Grunert P, Leite dos Santos A, et al. Symptomatic cysts of the cavum septi pellucidi and cavum vergae: the role of endoscopic neurosurgery in the treatment of four consecutive cases. Minim Invasive Neurosurg. 2003;46(4):243-9.

9. Sener RN. Cysts of the septum pellucidum. Comput Med Imaging Graph. 1995;19(4):357-60.

10. Heiskanen O. Cyst of the septum pellucidum causing increased intracranial pressure and hydrocephalus. Case report. J Neurosurg. 1973;38(6):771-3.

11. Van Wagenen WP, Aird RB. Dilatations of the cavity of the septum pellucidum and cavum vergae: report of cases. Am J Cancer. 1934;20(3):539-57.

12. Hughes RA, Kernohan JW, Craig WK. Caves and cysts of the septum pellucidum. AMA Arch Neurol Psychiatry. 1955;74(3):259-66.

13. Lancon JA, Haines DE, Raila FA, et al. Expanding cyst of the septum pellucidum. Case report. J Neurosurg. 1996;85(6):1127-34.

14. Aoki N. Cyst of the septum pellucidum presenting as hemiparesis. Childs Nerv Syst. 1986;2(6):326-8.

15. Borha A, Ponte KF, Emery E. Cavum septum pellucidum cyst in children: a case-based update. Childs Nerv Syst. 2012;28(6):813-9.

16. Gubbay SS, Vaughan R, Lekias JS. Intermittent hydrocephalus due to cysts of the septum pellucidum: a study of three cases. Clin Experiment Neurol. 1977;14:93-9.

17. Mapstone TB, White RJ. Cavum septi pellucidi as a cause of shunt dysfunction. Surg Neurol. 1981;16(2):96-8.

18. Hicdonmez T, Turan Suslu H, Butuc R, et al. Treatment of a large and symptomatic septum pellucidum cyst with endoscopic fenestration in a child—case report and review of the literature. Clin Neurol Neurosurg. 2012;114(7):1052-6.

19. Jackowski A, Kulshresta M, Sgouros S. Laser-assisted flexible endoscopic fenestration of giant cyst of the septum pellucidum. Br J Neurosurg. 1995;9(4):527-31.

20. Lancon JA, Haines DE, Lewis AI, et al. Endoscopic treatment of symptomatic septum pellucidum cysts: with some preliminary observations on the ultrastructure of the cyst wall: two technical case reports. Neurosurgery. 1999;45(5):1251-7.

21. Fratzoglou M, Leite dos Santos AR, Gawish I, et al. Endoscope-assisted microsurgery for tumors of the septum pellucidum: surgical considerations and benefits of the method in the treatment of four serial cases. Neurosurg Rev. 2005;28(1):39-43.

22. Miki T, Wada J, Nakajima N, et al. Operative indications and neuroendoscopic management of symptomatic cysts of the septum pellucidum. Childs Nerv Syst. 2005;21(5):372-81.

23. Meng H, Feng H, Le F, et al. Neuroendoscopic management of symptomatic septum pellucidum cysts. Neurosurgery. 2006;59(2):278-83; discussion 278-83.

24. Chiu CD, Huang WC, Huang MC, et al. Navigator system-assisted endoscopic fenestration of a symptomatic cyst in the septum pellucidum—technique and cases report. Clin Neurol Neurosurg. 2005;107(4):337-41.

25. Weyerbrock A, Mainprize T, Rutka JT. Endoscopic fenestration of a symptomatic cavum septum pellucidum: technical case report. Neurosurgery. 2006;59(4 Suppl 2):ONSE491; discussion ONSE.

26. Gangemi M, Maiuri F, Colella G, et al. Endoscopic surgery for intracranial cerebrospinal fluid cyst malformations. Neurosurg Focus. 1999;6(4):e6.

27. Gangemi M, Maiuri F, Cappabianca P, et al. Endoscopic fenestration of symptomatic septum pellucidum cysts: three case reports with discussion on the approaches and technique. Minim Invasive Neurosurg. 2002;45(2):105-8.

28. Roth J, Olasunkanmi A, Rubinson K, et al. Septal vein symmetry: implications for endoscopic septum pellucidotomy. Neurosurgery. 2010;67(2 Suppl Operative):395-401.

29. Akiyama K, Sato M, Sora I, et al. [A study of incidence and symptoms in 71 patients with cavum septi pellucidi]. No To Shinkei. 1983;35(6):575-81.

30. Flashman LA, Roth RM, Pixley HS, et al. Cavum septum pellucidum in schizophrenia: clinical and neuropsychological correlates. Psychiat Res. 2007;154(2):147-55.

31. Wester K, Krakenes J, Moen G. Expanding cava septi pellucidi and cava vergae in children: report of three cases. Neurosurgery. 1995;37(1):134-7.

CHAPTER 7

Arachnoid Cysts

David F Jimenez, Kevin R Carr

INTRODUCTION

Overall, arachnoid cysts of the cranial cavity are relatively common in the general population, with most being asymptomatic. When treatment is need either an open approach or shunting have been the primary treatment modalities. Endoscopic fenestration of symptomic arachnoid cysts provides the patient and surgeon with an easier, less invasive treatment option. This chapter describes how to manage these lesions and provides relevant clinical samples.

BACKGROUND

Arachnoid cysts are amorphous cystic cavities filled by a fluid mixture similar in composition to cerebrospinal fluid (CSF) that may present with signs associated with mass effect.[1,2] Primary cysts are most often described and are thought to be congenital abnormalities and though their existence has long since been known, their development is still debated. Some authors consider them a result of either malformations of the arachnoid mater or as a result of partial temporal lobe agenesis.[3,4] Earlier studies by Go and colleagues demonstrated that the cyst wall is lined with microvilli containing K-NPPase and alkaline phosphatase.[5] The enzymatic by-products are deposited into the cavity, consequently causing chronic expansion of the cyst cavity. Similar reports by Hellan and Associates support the notion that this enlargement and subsequent clinical presentations are due to secretory moieties associated with the luminal surface.[6] Their studies, however, supported a role for the NKCC1 cotransporter, which lines the luminal surface, in the enlargement of arachnoid

cysts by way of active secretion.[6] On the contrary, secondary arachnoid cysts are commonly called leptomeningeal cysts and typically arise as a result of traumatic brain injury or as a complication of prior surgery.[7-9] The ensuing arachnoiditis and inflammatory reactions allow for the accumulation of CSF between the leaflets of the arachnoid mater resulting in a dilated cavity.

While generally considered to be composed of arachnoid mater, studies have demonstrated that the constitution of the cyst wall is more variegated than initially thought of. In microscopic analysis of cysts excised from 24 patients, researchers in Sweden identified that 50% showed histologic variations from normal arachnoid and were comprised of a mixture of ciliated epithelia, simple epithelia, and fibrosis.[10] This may be important embryologically, as it suggests that this dysmorphology may have originated early in embryonic development. Clinically, this finding may not affect patient's outcome as no significant differences have been associated with the various cyst types and proclivity to cause mass effect.

CYST LOCATION

These lesions are typically supratentorial and approximately 50% to 66% are located in the middle cranial fossa abutting the adjacent temporal lobe (Figs. 1A to E).[11] Galassi and colleagues, in their edict, classified temporal fossa arachnoid cysts into three types based on their size and predilection for clinical complications.[12] Types II and III lesions occupy increasing portions of the temporal fossa with moderate to severe mass effect, respectively.[12] Consequently, patients present with chronic headaches,

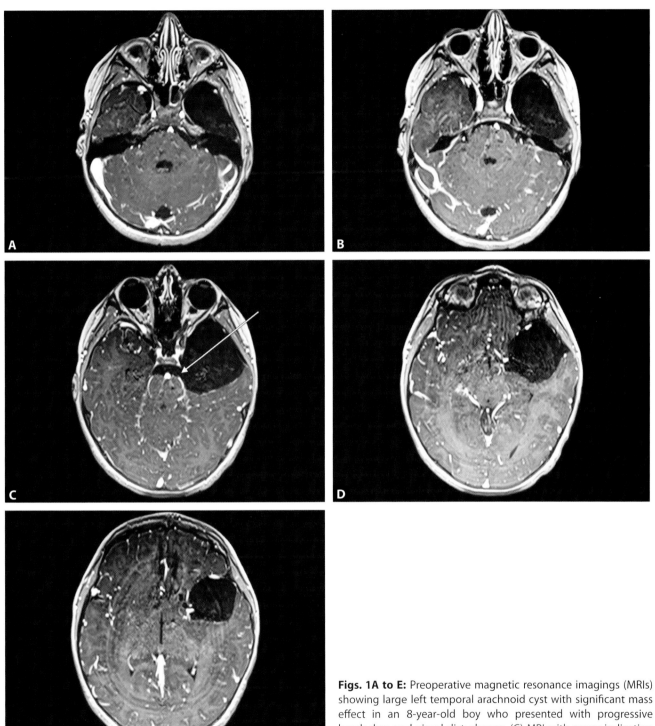

Figs. 1A to E: Preoperative magnetic resonance imagings (MRIs) showing large left temporal arachnoid cyst with significant mass effect in an 8-year-old boy who presented with progressive headaches and visual disturbance. (C) MRI with arrow indicating the area where the fenestration was performed.

macrocrania, and seizures in children.[13] Clinically, 60% to 80% of all discovered primary cysts are thought to be symptomatic.[13-16] However, while the decision to intervene is clear in these cases, various approaches have been promoted with no clear demonstration of superiority of either technique.[17-25]

TREATMENT OPTIONS

Currently, endoscopic cystoventriculostomy and ventriculocystocisternostomy are emerging as the minimally invasive approach of choice to address this condition. Various authors have demonstrated good clinical outcomes, low complication profiles, and low rates of re-operation in both adult and pediatric populations.[26-30] In El-Ghandour's small retrospective cohort study, 83% of symptomatic patients improved postoperatively, while 75% had substantial reduction of cyst size on follow-up. In his approach, a burr craniotomy overlying the lesion is created and a rigid endoscope is advanced into the parenchyma toward the cyst under neuronavigation. The cystostomy is achieved under neuronavigation guidance with subsequent ventriculostomy into the lateral ventricle ipsilateral to the cyst.[30] Similarly, in a more expansive assay on the neuroendoscopic approach to intracranial cysts, surgeons in Germany demonstrated 100% clinical improvement for the treatment of supratentorial arachnoid cysts using either a flexible or rigid endoscope.[26]

The choice of endoscope varies based on surgeon's preference, but historically rigid endoscopes have provided better visibility. However, limited maneuverability can create technical challenges for the operator.[31,32] Many authors however propose that the angled lenses available for rigid endoscopes nullify this disadvantage by allowing the user visibility around corners that otherwise is not available for flexible endoscopes.[26] As it relates to usability, rigid endoscope units are equipped with bi- or tri-port systems allowing for two-handed operations, which may be of benefit to some users.

SURGICAL PROCEDURE

General Principles

The primary goal of treating arachnoid cysts is to create a fenestration on the internal wall of the cyst and allow communication of the cyst's fluid with the subarachnoid cisterns, where the fluid will be reabsorbed along with CSF (Figs. 2A to E). Given that middle fossa arachnoid cysts are the most common, that means fenestrating the cyst to the subarachnoid spaces surrounding the midbrain. This can be a challenging endeavor as the space for fenestration is small and surrounded by vascular and neural structures. The fenestration can be accomplished in a number of ways depending on surgeon's preference (Figs. 4 to 8). My personal choice is to use a laser to perform the fenestration. The use of an energy-based instrument is to cauterize the edges of the fenestration so as to prevent future closure of the ostomy. Bluntly making the fenestration leaves floating wall edges that can fuse with time leading to closure and failure. Whenever possible, a Fogarty balloon can be used to expand the ostomy. Irrigation through the endoscopes working channel can aid in opening the fenestration and arachnoidal adhesions, when present. In order to ascertain physiologic parameters, it is my preference to always measure the intracranial pressure (ICP) prior to fenestration. Following the burr hole and exposure of the cyst's outer wall, a small opening is made with a bovie and needle tip followed by the rapid insertion of the ventricular catheter into the cyst. The catheter is then attached to a manometer and the intracystic and ICP is monitored and recorded. If desired, compliance testing can be done prior to removing the ventricular catheter. The fenestration can also be made with a Bugby wire or a monopolar instrument tip, getting the same result as a laser.

MIDDLE FOSSA CYSTS

The patient is placed supine with the head rotated to the contralateral side and on a cerebellar horseshoe headrest. The ipsilateral malar eminence should be placed so that the zygomatic arch is parallel to the floor. The neck should not be flexed and in a neutral position, so that cerebral venous outflow is not obstructed (Fig. 3). If neuronavigation is available, the preoperative images are loaded on the image-guided station and an entry point is selected. The entrance site should be located in an area where the cyst wall comes in contact with the skull. A trajectory is selected that allows access to the medial cisterns surrounding the brainstem. The skin is prepped with povidone-iodine solution and a small strip of hair is clipped to expose the scalp. Once the cranium is exposed, a burr hole is made with a craniotome. The outer cyst membrane should now be visible as previously explained. A small opening is made with the needle tip bovie set at 15 watts. A ventricle catheter is inserted and the ICP is measured. Cyst fluid is collected and sent for analysis. A peel-away introducer is inserted into the cyst or endoscopic metal cannula and obturator. A rigid endoscope with working channels is introduced and the cyst is inspected. The anatomy is relatively straightforward and the incisura is easily identified.

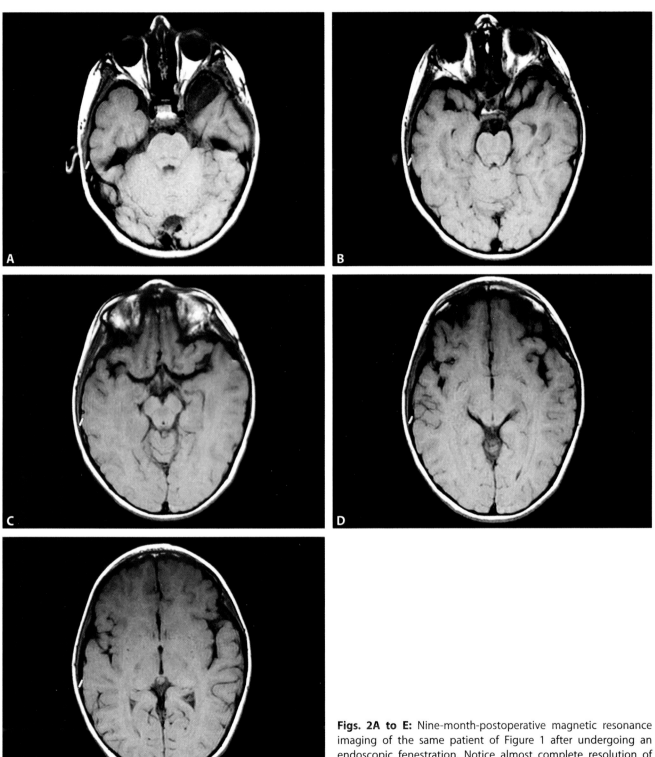

Figs. 2A to E: Nine-month-postoperative magnetic resonance imaging of the same patient of Figure 1 after undergoing an endoscopic fenestration. Notice almost complete resolution of the cyst and the patient had become asymptomatic. He continues to be asymptomatic 4 years postoperative.

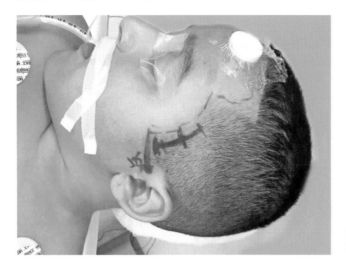

Fig. 3: Location of incision for fenestration of the patient in Figure 1.

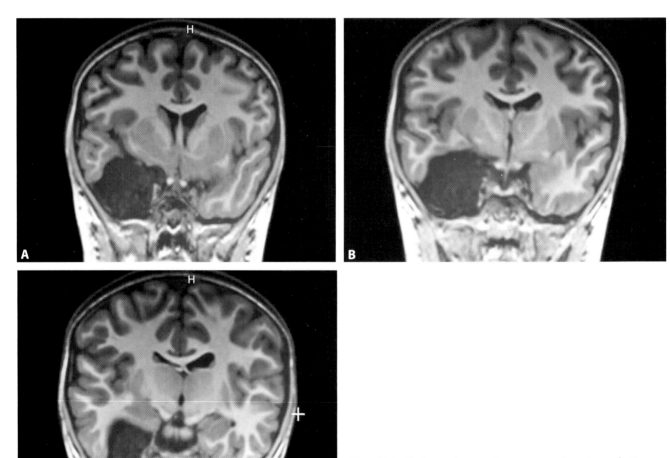

Figs. 4A to C: Coronal magnetic resonance imagings of a 7-year-old boy, who presented with headaches, nausea, and poor school performance. Scan shows large right middle fossa arachnoid cyst. Mass effect is seen on ipsilateral frontal horn.

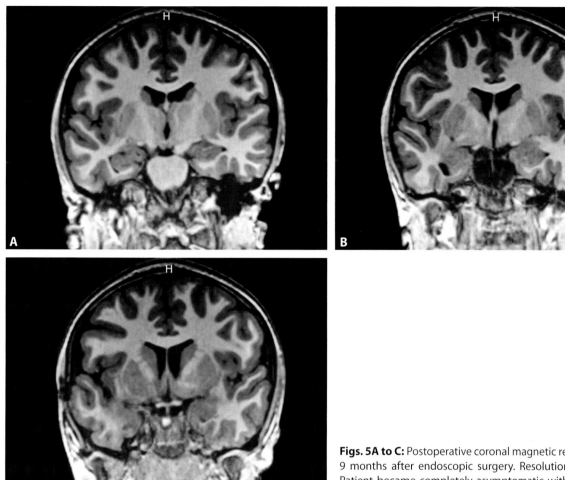

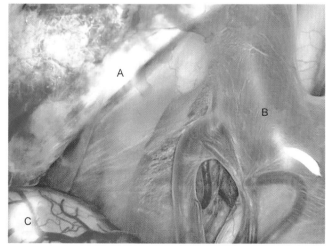

Figs. 5A to C: Postoperative coronal magnetic resonance imagings 9 months after endoscopic surgery. Resolution of cyst is noted. Patient became completely asymptomatic with improved school performance.

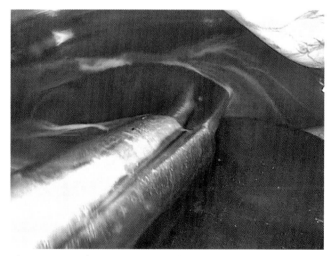

Fig. 6: Endoscopic view of patient with temporal arachnoid cyst. The incisura (A) is seen along with the middle cerebral artery (B) and the medial arachnoid membrane covering the basal cisterns around the temporal lobe (C).

Fig. 7: A pair of microscissors are being used to sharply cut and dissect the basal arachnoid membrane.

SUPRATENTORIAL AND CONVEXITY ARACHNOID CYSTS

Positioning

Once the neural, vascular, and bony landmarks are identified, the fenestration site is selected. The ostomy is performed with an energy source, as previously described, or with a blunt small probe or microscissors. Irrigation can be used to help open the ostomy and clear arachnoidal trabeculations. A Fogarty catheter can be used to expand the osteotomy if inspection reveals this to be a safe maneuver. The edges of the ostomy can be cauterized with the laser or bovie in order to minimize closure

of the ostomy. Closure is done with a standard fashion with placement of burr hole cover, subcutaneous closure, and skin closure with running nonabsorbable suture. The patient is monitored in hospital overnight and discharged the next day if clinically stable. Frontal (Figs. 9 and 10) and occipital cysts occur less frequently. However, positioning should maximize exposure to the cyst with a comfortable trajectory for the surgeon. Slight rotation of the head toward the operative side with shoulder rolls can maximize operator comfort for frontal lesions. To treat occipital and parietal lesions, a near recumbent posture can be assumed with occipital cups placed at the mastoids bilaterally.

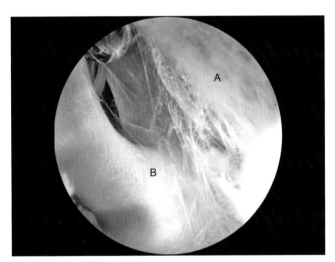

Fig. 8: After fenestration of the arachnoid membrane (A), the middle cerebral artery and (B) in the basal cistern are visualized on the left of the image.

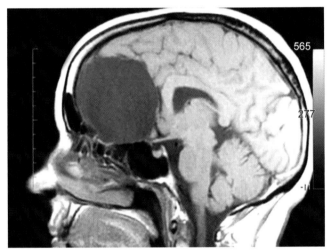

Fig. 9: Magnetic resonance imaging, sagittal view of very large frontal arachnoid cyst of a patient who presented with headaches and frontal lobe syndrome. Endoscopic fenestration was performed anterior to genu of corpus callosum.

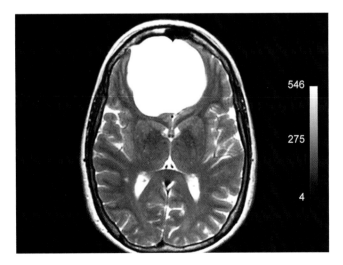

Fig. 10: Magnetic resonance imaging, axial view of same patient. Symptoms resolved after fenestration.

DEEP CEREBRAL AND INFRATENTORIAL ARACHNOID CYSTS

Though uncommon, there have been reports of arachnoid cysts located in proximity to the basal cisterns and deep cerebral structures. Understandably, these lesions are often juxtaposed to central CSF conduits, and expansion can cause rapidly symptomatic hydrocephalus. Of these, quadrigeminal arachnoid cysts are most often described and account for approximately 5% to 10% of intracranial arachnoid cysts.[30,33-35] Most quadrigeminal cysts are described in close approximation to the lateral or third ventricle. Cinalli described ventriculocystostomy of these lesions with either the lateral or third ventricle, or both to the intervening arachnoid cyst with good results.[35] In considering quadrigeminal cysts, whose walls abut the medial border of the lateral ventricle, they describe creating an initial ventriculostomy of the ipsilateral ventricle and subsequent cystostomy to the adjacent lesion. Care must be taken to avoid the internal cerebral veins which run in close proximity. They note preoperative vascular imaging to appreciate their course.[35] In lesions associated with the third ventricle, an endoscopic third ventriculostomy can also be completed to maximize decompression of the cyst. The management of the fenestration is done in a similar fashion as described in the section dealing with middle fossa arachnoid cysts. Another group of symptomatic arachnoid cysts includes these located in the posterior fossa and behind the cerebellum (Figs. 11 and 12). Successful fenestration may be accomplished via an endoscopic fenestration and a wide arachnoid cyst fenestration (Figs. 13 and 14).

CLINICAL CASE: MIDDLE FOSSA

The patient is a 4-year-old male who presented with a 2-year history of worsening headaches and increasingly more aggressive behavior. Although the headaches were global in nature, he consistently pointed to the right temporal area. On physical examination, there were no abnormalities in his general or neurologic exam. A diagnostic workup with brain CTs and MRIs (Figs. 15 to 17) demonstrated a progressively enlarging lesion consistent with an arachnoid cyst. A decision was made to take him to surgery to perform an endoscopic assisted fenestration of the lesion which was positively identified as an arachnoid cyst. An image guided approach was used and the lesion approach with an expanded burr hole (Figs. 18 to 21). The cyst was successfully fenestrated into the basal cisterns (Figs. 22A to C) and the patient's symptoms resolved.

CONCLUSION

Treatment of symptomatic arachnoid cysts can be done safely and effectively using endoscopic techniques. Once the surgeon has gained sufficient experience, these cases

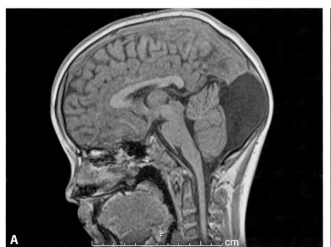
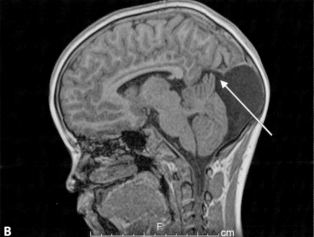

Figs. 11A and B: (A) A twelve-year-old boy presented with a large posterior fossa arachnoid cyst. Mid-sagittal noncontrast magnetic resonance imaging shows lesion placing significant mass effect on brainstem and cerebellum. (B) The cyst was approached endoscopically and the white arrow indicates the endoscope trajectory toward the site of fenestration.

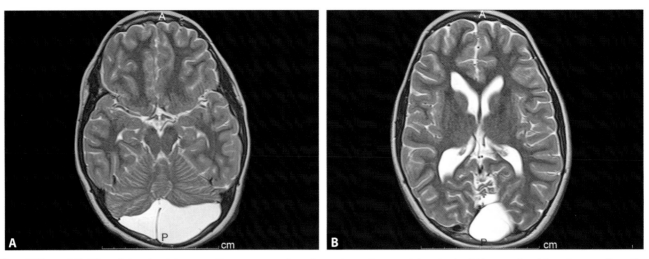

Figs. 12A and B: T2-weighted axial magnetic resonance imagings show the cranial extent of the arachnoid cyst as well as the compression of the cerebellum.

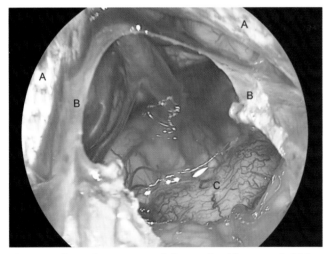

Fig. 13: A large fenestration of the arachnoid cyst wall (B) has been made. The dura of the tentorum is seen (A) as well as the compressed cerebellum (C).

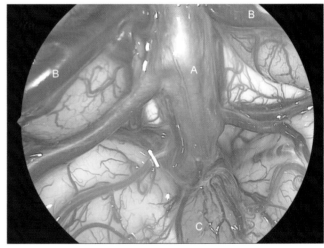

Fig. 14: Close-up endoscopic view of basal cisterns exposed. Notice the basal veins (B), the vein of Galen (A) and cerebellum (C).

can be done quickly (30–45 minutes) and efficiently. As the literature reports and in my own personal experience, a successful outcome can be achieved in up to 85% of the patients if the ostomy is properly performed. If the patient fails, a re-exploration is in order and if the ostomy is closed, a refenestration can be tried again, making sure that the opening is wide enough. If failure once again occurs, the cyst can be shunted to the peritoneal cavity. Endoscopic techniques in treating this condition can be valuable and useful tools for the treating surgeons.

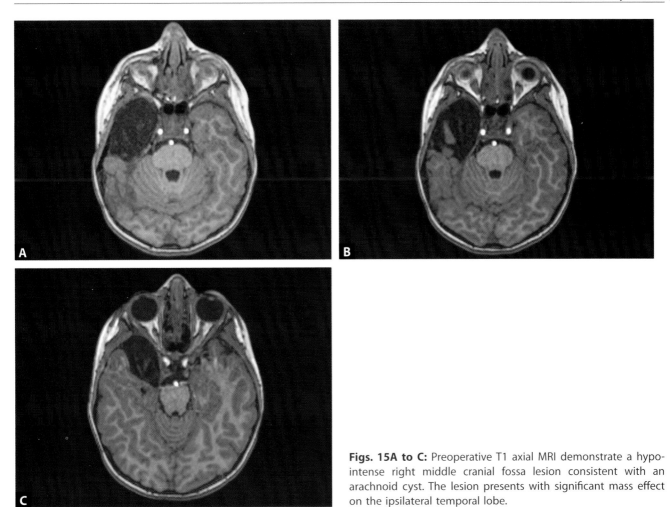

Figs. 15A to C: Preoperative T1 axial MRI demonstrate a hypo-intense right middle cranial fossa lesion consistent with an arachnoid cyst. The lesion presents with significant mass effect on the ipsilateral temporal lobe.

31.8 mm

Figs. 16A and B: Preoperative coronal MRI shows cyst elevation and compression of the inferior temporal lobe.

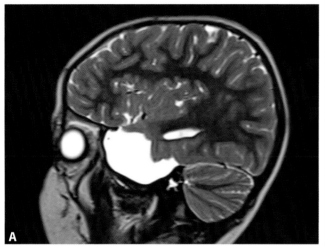
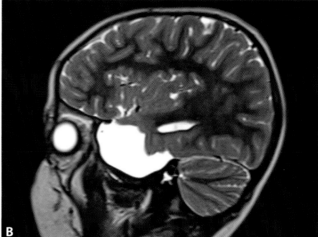

Figs. 17A and B: Preoperative T2 sagittal MRI depicts a hyperintense area consistent with CSF and an arachnoid cyst.

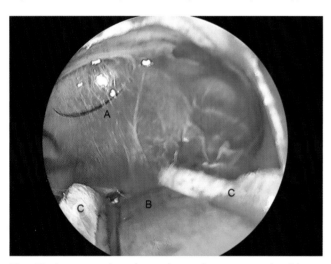
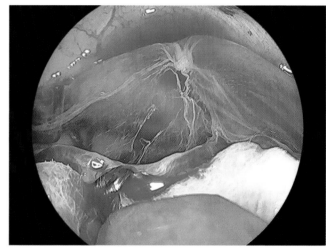

Fig. 18: Intraoperative photo shows the outer arachnoid cyst wall (A) in the middle temporal fossa. The temporal lobe is being gently retracted with a brain ribbon (B) and cottonoid patties (C).

Fig. 19: The outer cyst wall has been fenestrated and the cyst decompressed. A superficial temporal lobe vein is seen distal to the end of the brain ribbon retractor.

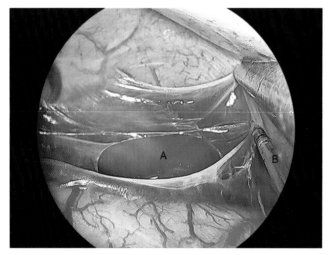
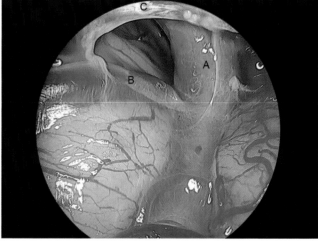

Fig. 20: The fenestration (A) is being enlarged and the cyst wall fulgurated with a GOLD laser microfiber (B).

Fig. 21: The cyst has been fenestrated into the basal cistern between the main trunk of the middle cerebral artery (A), one of the primary temporal branches (B) and the incisura (C).

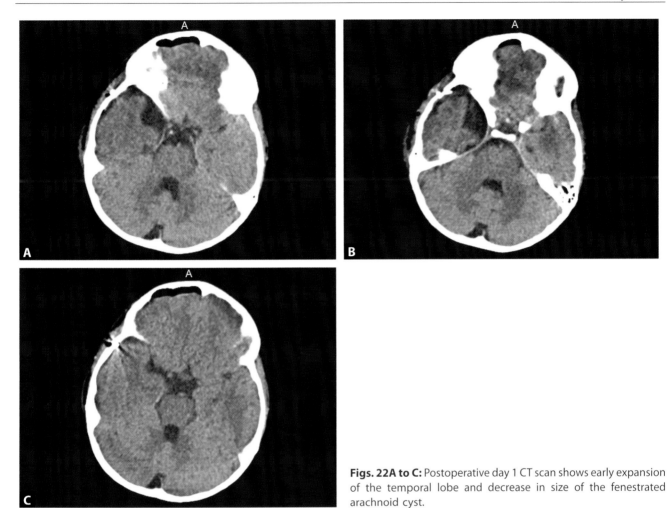

Figs. 22A to C: Postoperative day 1 CT scan shows early expansion of the temporal lobe and decrease in size of the fenestrated arachnoid cyst.

REFERENCES

1. Binitie O, Williams B, Case CP. A suprasellar subarachnoid pouch; aetiological considerations. J Neurol Neurosurg Psychiatry. 1984;47(10):1066-74.
2. Armstrong EA, Harwood-Nash DC, Hoffman H, et al. Benign suprasellar cysts: the CT approach. AJNR Am J Neuroradiol. 1983;4:163-6.
3. Robinson RG. The temporal lobe agenesis syndrome. Brain. 1964;87:87-106.
4. Starkman SP, Brown TC, Linell EA. Cerebral arachnoid cysts. J Neuropathol Exp Neurol. 1958;17:484-500.
5. Go KG, Houthoff HJ, Blaauw EH, et al. Arachnoid cysts of the sylvian fissure. Evidence of fluid secretion. J Neurosurg. 1984;60:803-13.
6. Helland CA, Aarhus M, Knappskog P, et al. Increased NKCC1 expression in arachnoid cysts supports secretory basis for cyst formation. Exp Neurol. 2010;224:424-8.
7. Ruscalleda J, Guardia E, dos Santos FM, et al. Dynamic study of arachnoid cysts with metrizamide. Neuroradiology. 1980;20:185-9.
8. Schachenmayr W, Friede RL. Fine structure of arachnoid cysts. J Neuropathol Exp Neurol. 1979;38:434-46.
9. Taveras JM, Ransohoff J. Leptomeningeal cysts of the brain following trauma with erosion of the skull; a study of seven cases treated by surgery. J Neurosurg. 1953;10:233-41.
10. Rabiei K, Tisell M, Wikkelso C, et al. Diverse arachnoid cyst morphology indicates different pathophysiological origins. Fluids Barriers CNS. 2014;11(1):5.
11. Robertson SJ, Wolpert SM, Runge VM. MR imaging of middle cranial fossa arachnoid cysts: temporal lobe agenesis syndrome revisited. AJNR Am J Neuroradiol. 1989; 10:1007-10.
12. Galassi E, Tognetti F, Gaist G, et al. CT scan and metrizamide CT cisternography in arachnoid cysts of the middle cranial fossa: classification and pathophysiological aspects. Surg Neurol. 1982;17:363-9.
13. Locatelli D, Bonfanti N, Sfogliarini R, et al. Arachnoid cysts: diagnosis and treatment. Child's Nerv Syst. 1987; 3:121-4.

14. Sato K, Shimoji T, Yaguchi K, et al. Middle fossa arachnoid cyst: clinical, neuroradiological, and surgical features. Child's Brain. 1983;10:301-16.

15. Harsh GR 4th, Edwards MS, Wilson CB. Intracranial arachnoid cysts in children. J Neurosurg. 1986;64:835-42.

16. Galassi E, Piazza G, Gaist G, et al. Arachnoid cysts of the middle cranial fossa: a clinical and radiological study of 25 cases treated surgically. Surg Neurol. 1980;14:211-9.

17. Pierre-Kahn A, Capelle L, Brauner R, et al. Presentation and management of suprasellar arachnoid cysts. Review of 20 cases. J Neurosurg. 1990;73:355-9.

18. Sato H, Sato N, Katayama S, et al. Effective shunt-independent treatment for primary middle fossa arachnoid cyst. Child's Nerv Syst. 1991;7:375-81.

19. Pell MF, Thomas DG. The management of infratentorial arachnoid cyst by CT-directed stereotactic aspiration. Br J Neurosurg. 1991;5:399-403.

20. Oberbauer RW, Haase J, Pucher R. Arachnoid cysts in children: a European co-operative study. Child's Nerv Syst. 1992;8:281-6.

21. Kurokawa Y, Sohma T, Tsuchita H, et al. A case of intraventricular arachnoid cyst. How should it be treated? Child's Nerv Syst. 1990;6:365-7.

22. Iacono RP, Labadie EL, Johnstone SJ, et al. Symptomatic arachnoid cyst at the clivus drained stereotactically through the vertex. Neurosurgery. 1990;27:130-3.

23. Dei-Anang K, Voth D. Cerebral arachnoid cyst: a lesion of the child's brain. Neurosurg Rev. 1989;12:59-62.

24. Barth A, Seiler RW. Surgical treatment of suprasellar arachnoid cyst. Eur Neurol. 1994;34:51-2.

25. Artico M, Cervoni L, Salvati M, et al. Supratentorial arachnoid cysts: clinical and therapeutic remarks on 46 cases. Acta Neurochir. 1995;132:75-8.

26. Tirakotai W, Schulte DM, Bauer BL, et al. Neuroendoscopic surgery of intracranial cysts in adults. Child's Nerv Syst. 2004;20:842-51.

27. Sengul G, Tuzun Y, Cakir M, et al. Neuroendoscopic approach to quadrigeminal cistern arachnoid cysts. Eurasian J Med. 2012;44:18-21.

28. Giannetti AV, Fraga SM, Silva MC, et al. Endoscopic treatment of interhemispheric arachnoid cysts. Pediat Neurosurg. 2012;48:157-62.

29. Schroeder HW, Gaab MR, Niendorf WR. Neuroendoscopic approach to arachnoid cysts. J Neurosurg. 1996;85:293-8.

30. El-Ghandour NM. Endoscopic treatment of intraparenchymal arachnoid cysts in children. J Neurosurg. Pediatrics. 2014;14:501-7.

31. Carr K, Zuckerman SL, Tomycz L, et al. Endoscopic removal of an intraventricular primitive neuroectodermal tumor: retrieval of a free-floating fragment using a urological basket retriever. J Neurosurg Pediatrics. 2013;12:25-9.

32. Grondin RT, Hader W, MacRae ME, et al. Endoscopic versus microsurgical resection of third ventricle colloid cysts. Can J Neurol Sci. 2007;34:197-207.

33. Gangemi M, Maiuri F, Colella G, et al. Endoscopic treatment of quadrigeminal cistern arachnoid cysts. Minim Invasive Neurosurg. 2005;48:289-92.

34. Inamasu J, Ohira T, Nakamura Y, et al. Endoscopic ventriculo-cystomy for non-communicating hydrocephalus secondary to quadrigeminal cistern arachnoid cyst. Acta Neurol Scand. 2003;107:67-71.

35. Cinalli G, Spennato P, Columbano L, et al. Neuroendoscopic treatment of arachnoid cysts of the quadrigeminal cistern: a series of 14 cases. J Neurosurg Pediatrics. 2010;6:489-97.

CHAPTER 8

Endoscopic Management of Frontal Epidural Lesions

David F Jimenez

INTRODUCTION

Lesions commonly present in the epidural space throughout the cranium which may become symptomatic and require treatment or are unknown and require diagnosis. Epidural lesions located in the frontal and frontotemporal areas require close attention to both treatment as well as cosmesis related to the approach. Typically and in order not to leave scars on the face or forehead, a bicoronal scalp incision is necessary along with marked scalp mobilization and subsequent swelling, bruising, and discomfort. The author has successfully used endoscopic-based techniques to reach low or mid frontal areas with excellent result and minimal associated trauma. Presented herein are cases and techniques to accomplish such an approach.

POSITIONING

The patient is induced under general anesthesia either using endotracheal intubation or a laryngeal mask airway. The selection site for the scalp incision is made behind the hairline and on the side of the lesion. The patient's head, forehead, and face are prepped with a povidone-iodine solution. Corneal protectors are used with lubricating ophthalmic ointment. The head is placed on a cerebellar horseshoe type head holder and is freely moveable throughout the procedure. Intravenous antibiotics are given in a standard fashion prior to skin incision.

INCISION

A 3-cm incision is made behind the hairline after a small amount of hair has been clipped. Monopolar dissection of the dermis, subcutaneous tissues, and galea can be done bloodlessly with a needle tip attachment. The location should be placed so that there is direct access to the lesion with the shortest distance. The pericranium is incised and reflected to expose the cranium in preparation for the burr hole.

CRANIAL ACCESS

These lesions can be easily approached via a single burr hole using a craniotomy or a hand drill. A standard adult size ACRA-CUT® (ACRA-CUT, Inc. Acton, MA) bit is used to make the burr hole. This system leaves a small shelf of bone which needs to be removed with Kerrison Rongeurs. As the hole is made directly perpendicular to the skull, the opening to the dura has the same trajectory (Fig. 1). However, the lesion needs to be approached at an angle. Likewise, Kerrison Rongeurs (or a match stick drill bit) are used to undercut the base of the burr hole and to aid with the passage of the endoscope (Fig. 2). This maneuver significantly increases the working area where the endoscope and adjunct instruments can be placed.

PROCEDURE

Either a rigid or flexible endoscope can be used depending on the location of the lesion. The flexible endoscope provides for increased maneuverability and minimizes the amount of dural retraction needed to reach the lesion. Once the burr hole has been appropriately sized, the flexible endoscope can be placed over the dura and advanced toward the lesions. Ongoing irrigation may be used or needed to develop an epidural place and increase the working surface area (Fig. 3). Because the endoscope can be manipulated, it

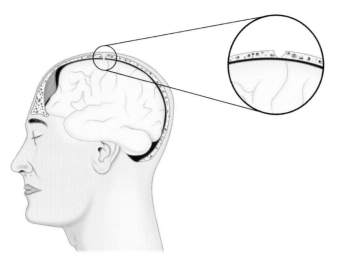

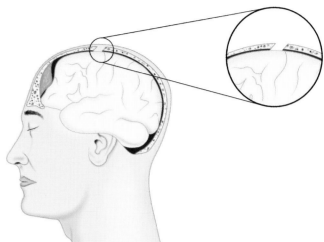

Fig. 1: Artistic diagram shows frontal location of lesion. The endoscopic approach is via a posterior frontal burr hole placed behind the hairline. A standard craniotome creates a burr hole with a small shelf of inner skull table at the bottom of hole as seen in expanded figure.

Fig. 2: Kerrison Rongeur or a match stick drill bit can be used to undercut the frontal aspect of the burr hole and uppercut the parietal aspect of the burr hole. This maneuver angulates the burr hole and its trajectory toward the lesion.

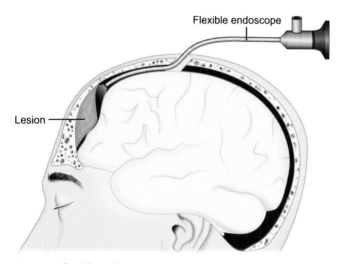

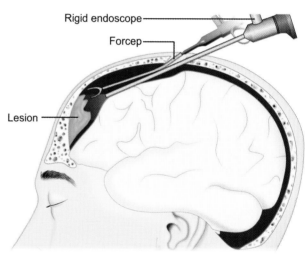

Fig. 3: A flexible endoscope can then be passed and advanced toward the low lying frontal lesion over the frontal convexity and dura.

Fig. 4: A flexible or rigid endoscope can be advanced fronto-inferiorly to reach the lesion. If a hematoma is present, forceps can be used to break the clot and suction/irrigation used for complete evacuation.

is advanced curving around the frontal convexity. A malleable suction tip can be used, both as a dissector as well as a suction instrument. Both the endoscope and suction tip are advance toward the lesion in tandem.

Once the lesion is visible, biopsies can be taken with biopsy forceps (Fig. 4) and sent to the laboratory for proper identification. If a hematoma is present it may be broken up with forceful irrigation and suction. Both the endoscope and the flexible suction tip can be advanced so that the entire lesion may be removed. If an abscess is present, cultures

and liquid aspiration can be done so that samples can be sent to the lab. The abscess can then be fully evacuated using irrigation and suction the entire surgical field can be inspected and the surgeon makes sure that the lesion has been totally and satisfactorily removed. The instruments are removed and a titanium burr hole cover is placed over the cranial opening. The galea and skin are closed in standard fashion. The patient may be discharged to home or observed overnight in the hospital.

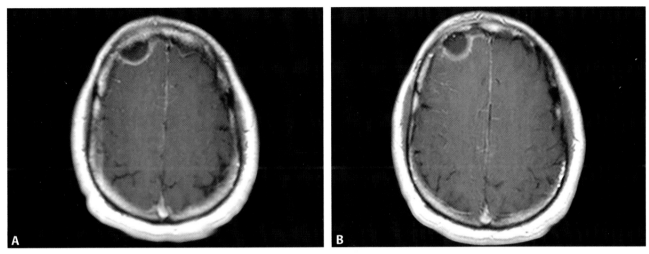

Figs. 5A and B: Axial T$_1$ postgadolinium contrast magnetic resonance imagings done preoperative demonstrate a right frontal hypointense lesion with ring enhancement consistent with an infectious process.

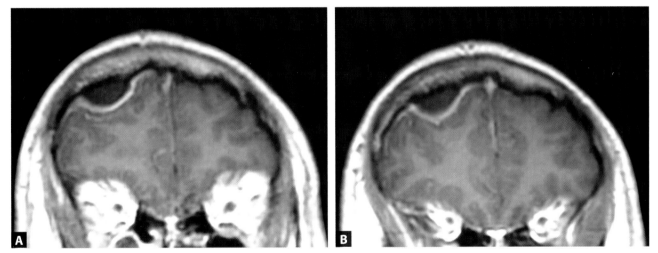

Figs. 6A and B: Preoperative coronal contrasted magnetic resonance imagings show the hypointense lesion with ring enhancement.

CLINICAL CASES

Case 1

Forty-three-year-old right-handed male presented with a history of chronic headaches and previously treated bouts of sinusitis. The patient had severe frontal headaches, fever (T$_{max}$ 101.9°F), nausea, and fatigue. Diagnostic work up with computed tomography (CT) scans and magnetic resonance imaging (MRI) scans (Figs. 5 to 7) demonstrated an extra axial hypointense right-sided lesion whose rim enhanced following the administration of gadolinium intravenously. The lesion was consistent with an epidural abscess. A decision was made to treat and diagnose the lesion. The patient agreed to an endoscopic approach. He was taken to the operating room (OR) where, under general anesthesia, an endoscopic approach was undertaken. The lesion was approached via a small 14 mm burr hole placed along the mid pupillary line and behind the hairline on the right side (Fig. 8). The edges of the burr hole were expanded as shown in Figure 2 exposing the dura (Fig. 9). Flexible endoscope was advanced frontoinferiorly and a yellowish, creamy mass was encountered. Gram stains showed a gram positive bacterium. Using irrigation and suction, the lesion was fully evacuated. The patient was placed on the appropriate antibiotics. One week after surgery the patient's CT scans showed

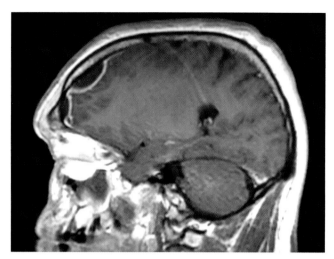

Fig. 7: Sagittal preoperative magnetic resonance imaging shows several epidural rim enhancing lesions with a hypointense center consistent with an epidural abscess.

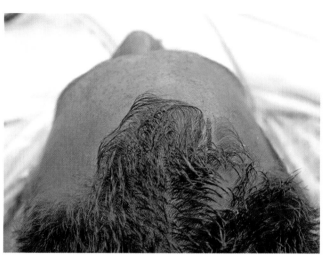

Fig. 8: Intraoperative photograph of patient resting on cerebellar head rest. The proposed incision has been marked and is located along the mid pupillary line on the right side.

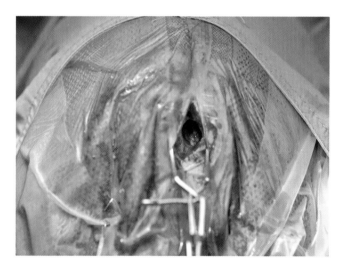

Fig. 9: Burr hole has been made and carefully expanded antereoinferiorly to allow endoscopic access to the lesion.

complete resolution of the abscess (Figs. 10A to C) and was afebrile and headache free and follow up at 3 months, the patient remained symptom free.

Case 2

Twenty-one-year-old male was assaulted on a Saturday night. The next day he woke up with severe frontal headaches and went to an outside hospital where a CT scan was obtained which showed a small right frontal epidural hematoma. His symptoms progressed and on repeat CT scan (Figs. 11A and B), the epidural was seen enlarging. The patient was taken to the OR where a frontal endoscopic approach was undertaken. The hematoma was removed with irrigation, forceps, and suction. SURGIFLO® (Ethicon, Somerville, NJ) was left on the surgical site. The patient tolerated the procedure well. On follow-up CT scan (postoperative day 1) the hematoma was seen to be evacuated (Figs. 12A and B). A repeat CT scan on postoperativeday 10 (Figs. 13A and B) showed marked resolution of the hematoma. He was last seen on follow-up 3 months later and was back to work and completely asymptomatic.

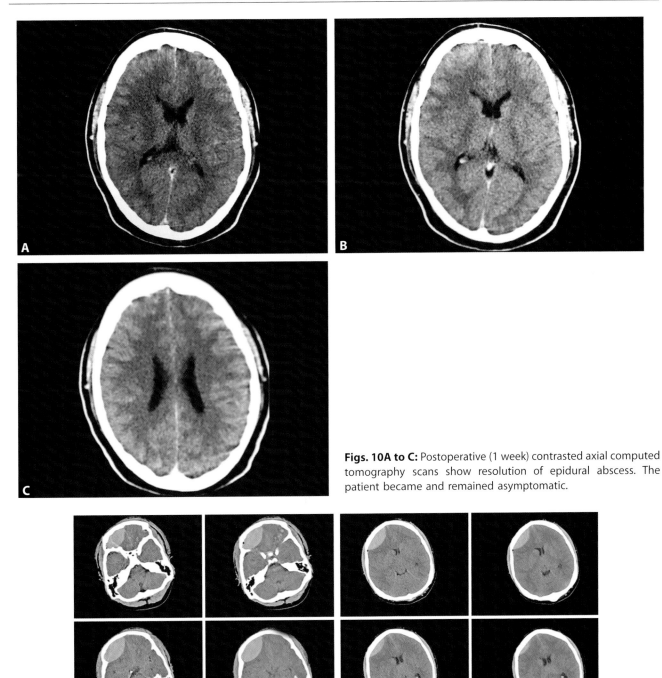

Figs. 10A to C: Postoperative (1 week) contrasted axial computed tomography scans show resolution of epidural abscess. The patient became and remained asymptomatic.

Figs. 11A and B: Preoperative computed tomography scans show large right frontal epidural hematoma with a mass effect in a symptomatic 26-year-old male.

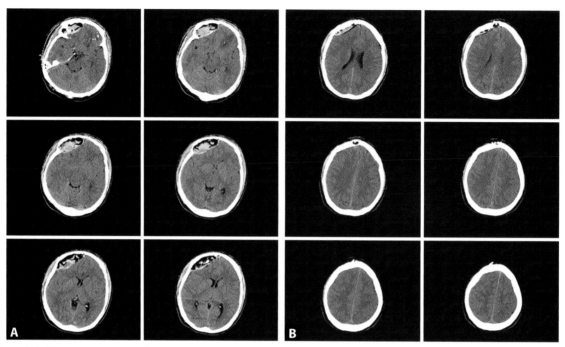

Figs. 12A and B: First postoperative day computed tomography scan shows significant evacuation of right epidural frontal lesion. Remaining SURGIFLO® represents low density area in the surgical site.

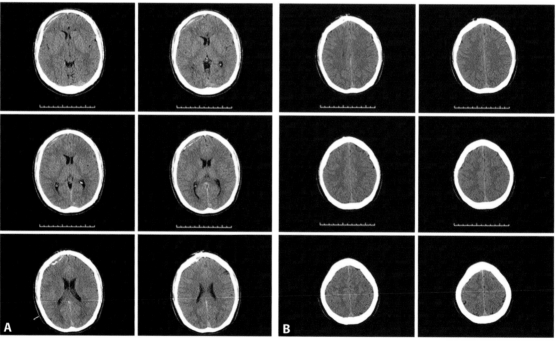

Figs. 13A and B: Computerized tomography scans done 10 days after endoscopic evacuation of hematoma demonstrate significant lesional resolution. Patient was symptom free.

CONCLUSION

Carefully selected unilateral frontal epidural lesions such as abscesses or hematomas may be successfully evacuated with the use of endoscopes and endoscopic techniques. This approach leads to excellent cosmetic result and less trauma to the patient.

CHAPTER 9

Endoscopic Resection of Colloid Cysts

David F Jimenez, David N Garza

INTRODUCTION

Colloid cysts are benign, thin-walled, spherical neoplasms composed of a collagenous capsule, an underlying epithelium, and a viscous center.[1] They represent approximately 1% of all intracranial neoplasms, 15% to 20% of all intraventricular tumors, and have an estimated yearly incidence of 3.2 per 1,000,000.[2-4] Large colloid cysts are rare. Most reported cases do not exceed 3 cm, but 5 cm and 8 cm cysts have been documented.[5] Patients with colloid cysts may present with symptoms such as chronic or acute headaches, nausea, vomiting, drowsiness, memory loss, gait abnormality, incontinence, disorders of consciousness, and psychiatric symptoms.[3,6,7]

Because the clinical presentation is so diverse, the only way to confirm the presence of a colloid cyst is through diagnostic imaging, such as computerized tomography and/or magnetic resonance imaging (MRI).[6]

Colloid cysts are usually located within the rostral part of the third ventricle near the foramina of Monro, between the columns of the fornix[8] (Figs. 1 to 3). Their etiology has been the subject of much debate. It was once theorized that colloid cysts were remnants of the paraphysis or formed from detachments of developing neuroepithelium within the choroid plexus.[9-12] More contemporary evidence provided by immunohistochemical and ultrastructural studies suggests that the cysts actually have an

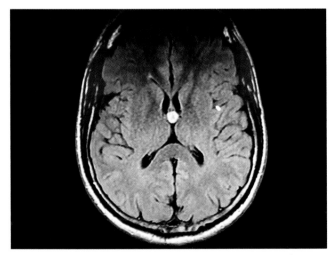

Fig. 1: MRI FLAIR, axial image at the level of foramen of Monro demonstrates a hyperintense round lesion behind the columns of the fornices consistent with a colloid cyst. (MRI: Magnetic resonance imaging; FLAIR: Fluid attenuation inversion recovery).

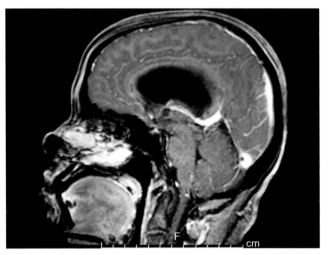

Fig. 2: Contrast T_1 sagittal magnetic resonance imaging shows a colloid cyst with an enhancing wall but nonenhancing cystic contents causing obstructive hydrocephalus.

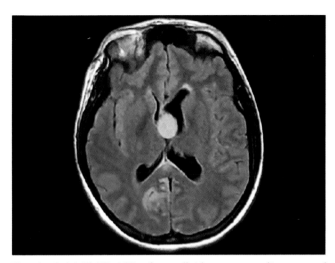

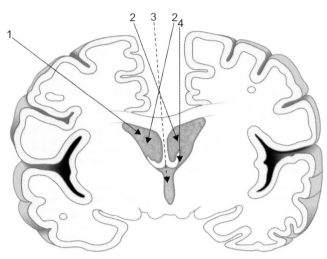

Fig. 3: Axial FLAIR MRI of a colloid cyst extending toward the left frontal horn and causing unilateral dilation of the left ventricular system. (FLAIR: Fluid attenuation inversion recovery; MRI: Magnetic resonance imaging).

Fig. 4: Diagram shows the various approaches used to reach and resect colloid cysts. Approach 1 is transcortical and can be endoscopic or open microsurgery. Approaches 2, 3, and 4 are variations of the transcallosal approach.

endodermal derivation.[13] Because endodermal elements are not normally present in the roof of the third ventricle, some authors speculate that colloid cyst histogenesis might be initiated by the migration of respiratory epithelial precursors into the velum interpositum during development.[10,13]

Several studies have determined that colloid cysts are composed of ciliated and nonciliated, cuboidal, pseudostratified or columnar epithelial cells interspersed with goblet cells that secrete amorphous, proteinaceous material.[14] As the patient ages, the gradual buildup of this secreted material forms colloid cysts. Although they are benign, the cysts can provoke acute deterioration or even cause sudden death if they cause obstructive hydrocephalus and increase a patient's ICP.[15,16] The definitive cause of this rapid deterioration is still not fully understood. Rickert et al. hypothesized that the acute blockage created by a cyst can cause a pressure-induced decompensation of cerebral neuronal pathways that disrupts the cardiopulmonary control centers in the reticular formation of the brain stem, which can led to instantaneous cardiorespiratory arrest.[17] In symptomatic patients, the risk for precipitous decline or death has been estimated to be as high as 34%.[15] Tumor size and the duration of symptoms do not appear to be reliable prognostic indicators of this dire outcome.[16]

Death can result if growth is sudden, but if the cyst enlarges gradually the patient's anatomy can accommodate the mass at the foramen of Monro without disrupting cerebrospinal fluid (CSF) flow, which would allow the patient to remain asymptomatic.[14] It has been estimated that between 40% and 50% of colloid cysts are asymptomatic.[5] Rather than undergoing immediate surgery, these patients can have serial neuroimaging performed in order to monitor their cyst's growth. If the cysts enlarge, hydrocephalus may develop, if the patient becomes symptomatic, then surgical intervention will become a necessary recourse to prevent neurological decline.[14] Because the size, content, composition, and density of colloid cysts are so diverse, they may have very different imaging appearances.[6] In 1933, Dandy published a monograph on benign tumors of the third ventricle and reported a 20% mortality rate for his surgical intervention.[18,19] Since that time, microsurgical and endoscopic techniques have drastically reduced patient mortality rates. Third ventricular colloid cysts are currently managed by either a transcallosal or transcortical craniotomy and resection or via an endoscopic approach through the frontal lobe[3,20] (Fig. 4). Microsurgery offers a higher rate of radical excision than endoscopy but often results in longer operative times and more frequent cognitive dysfunction.[3] Endoscopic approaches are generally associated with lower rates of morbidity and mortality; they frequently involve shorter hospital stays and a smaller risk for cognitive impairment.[3,21] Because they are less invasive, endoscopic approaches often have higher rates of patient satisfaction. In a study conducted by Sribnick et al., 92% of patients who had undergone endoscopic resection were able to return to work 4–5 weeks after surgery and 100% indicated that they were satisfied with their operations.[22] The primary goal of surgery is to open up the blocked foramina of Monro and establish CSF outflow so that obstructive hydrocephalus is treated. The ideal goal is complete removal of the cyst but, due to its very close relationship to the internal cerebral views and choroid plexus, hemorrhage presents as a likely and probable risk. When such risk is present, subtotal resection of the lesion should be considered with fulguration and coagulation of as much of the remaining capsule as possible. The patient can then be followed expectantly with serial MRIs.

Endoscopy provides multiple angles of visualization and superior illumination, but the operating surgeon must have experience with the technique and dexterity using both hands simultaneously in order for it to be effective.[3] With an experienced operator at the helm, an endoscopic approach can be considered the primary treatment for colloid cyst patients. However, because there is a chance residual cysts will remain after an endoscopic procedure, reoperation might be necessary to minimize the patient's risk for recurrence.[6,20] When evaluating the completeness of cyst resection, surgeons should use direct, intraoperative observation rather than relying solely on postoperative imaging. MRI is less sensitive in its capacity to detect cyst remnants, which ultimately makes it an ineffective tool for predicting recurrence.[23] A key step in endoscopic cyst resection is the identification of an entry point. An optimal entry point can facilitate the procedure, increase the chance for total resection, and aid in the preservation of key anatomical structures, such as the caudate nucleus, deep cerebral veins, and fornices.[24] However, there is a difference of opinion regarding where the optimal entry point is and which endoscopic approach is best to use under different anatomical circumstances.

ACCESS POINT

Early endoscopists used the traditional approach to the frontal horn by selecting Kocher's point which is defined as 1 cm anterior to the coronal suture and 3 cm lateral from the midline.[25] Although this entry point does allow access to the frontal horn, the senior author finds this access point to be significantly disadvantageous. The goal, when approaching a lesion located in the third ventricle from the frontal horn, is to have a direct and enface

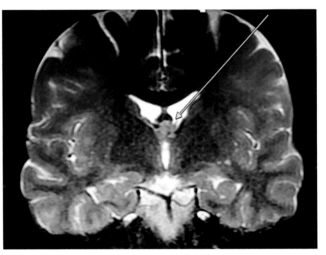

Fig. 5: T_2-weighted coronal magnetic resonance imaging with a colloid cyst. The yellow arrow indicates the preferred trajectory and lateral entry site. Care should be taken not to injure the head of the caudate nucleus.

view of the cyst. By using Kocher's point, the surgeon approaches the lesion from a superior point which makes it difficult to have direct access to the lesion. A 90° turn of the endoscope is needed to reach the cyst and work with it and as such the use of a rigid rod lens endoscope is precluded. Flexible endoscopes can be used but require significantly more surgeon's experience and maneuverability. The author preferred entry point is located laterally between 6 cm and 8 cm from the midline and near to the coronal suture. The exact location can be selected from the sagittal and coronal MRI images. The trajectory should take the access portal immediately superior to the head of the Caudate Nucleus and directly to the foramen of Monro (Fig. 5). If image guided navigation is available, then the entry target points can be selected in the operating room (Figs. 6 to 8).

POSITIONING

Once general anesthesia has been induced, the patient is placed supine on the operating room table. The head can be freely placed on a cerebellar horseshoe head holder or on a Mayfield type 3 point cranial fixation clamp (Fig. 9). It is the author's preference to use the latter. To have the patient's head inadvertently move while performing surgery can have devastating consequences. The head is placed in neutral position with relation to the floor. It may be slightly rotated to the contralateral side

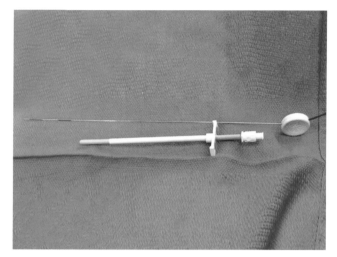

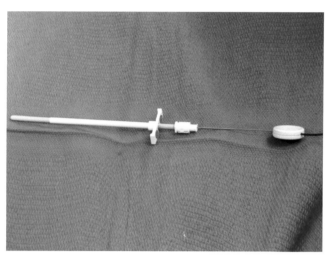

Fig. 6: The peel-away introducer consists of an outer cannula (white) and an obturator (blue). The cannula is 14 cm in length but is cut at 10 cm for greater accuracy. The image guided tracker is seen next to the introducer.

Fig. 7: The tracker is introduced inside the obturator so that its tip can be tracked in a triplanar fashion. Care is taken to advance the end of the white cannula to the tip of the obturator prior to insertion into the ventricle.

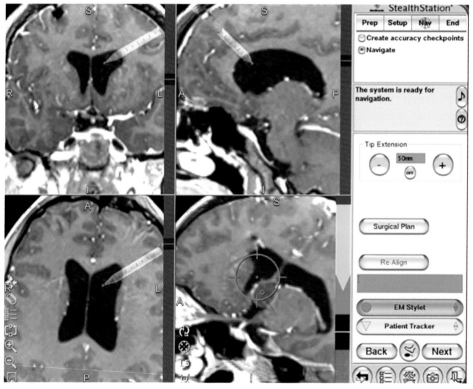

Fig. 8: Screenshot from stealth station navigation system. The proper trajectory to target can be seen in triplanar slices as well as the direct view to the lesion as seen in the right lower image.

by 5–10° if navigation is being used. Care is taken to make sure that cranial venous outflow is not restricted in any way. Ventilation is set to normocarbia and fluid intake to euvolemic.

INCISION AND ENTRY

Once the incision site is selected, a small strip of hair is clipped and the scalp is prepped with povidone-iodine

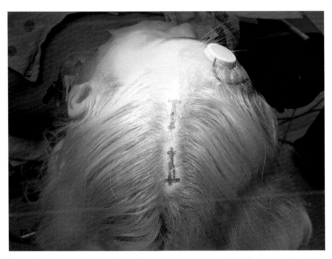

Fig. 9: Patient's position for endoscopic colloid cyst resection. The two portal approach is used and the hair has been clipped and two small incisions marked lateral to midline. The forehead navigation sensor is taped to the forehead.

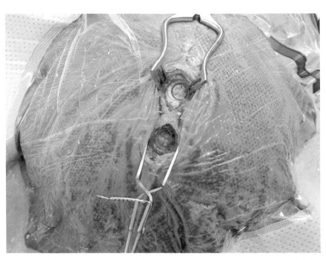

Fig. 10: The same patient has been prepped and two burr holes made showing the dura mater.

solution. If the hair is long, it can be secured in place with sponges or towels stapled to the scalp. Incision can be made with a monopolar needle tip set at 15 watts on cut mode. The pericranium is mobilized and the cranial bone exposed. The procedure can be safely done with a single burr hole; however, the author's preferred access is a biportal technique whereby two burr holes are made 6–8 cm lateral from the midline and at and in front of the coronal suture (Fig. 10). Adding a second portal enhances the surgeon's ability to manipulate and resect the lesion. The posterior portal can be used to introduce the endoscope with the working channels. The anterior burr hole can be used to place a Frazier type suction unit which can be used to aspirate the thick, gelatinous contents of the colloid cyst once the capsule is opened. In 2013, Wilson et al. agreed with our approach and described a dual-instrument anterolateral approach to endoscopic resection that placed the entry point 5 cm anterior to the coronal suture and 5–7 cm lateral to midline depending on the degree of ventriculomegaly present.[25] According to the authors, this new approach helped them reach the foramen of Monro perpendicularly, which preserved the fornix; their bimanual, dual-instrument technique helped apply tension to the cyst wall, used fewer side-to-side endoscope movements associated with trauma, and afforded the operators with a higher degree of surgical control.[25] Sribnick et al. affirmed some of these findings after conducting their own studies. They believed that the

anterolateral trajectory in conjunction with a 30° working channel endoscope enabled direct visualization of the fornix, the thalamostriate and septal veins and the arteriolar feeders to the colloid cyst capsule as well as the site of attachment of the cyst to the roof of the third ventricle.[22] Whenever possible image guided navigation should be used to improve accuracy and safety. The exact location of the peel-away introducer can be obtained by inserting the navigation tracker into the obturator working channel.

Procedure

Once the burr holes have been made and the dura mater exposed the needle tip bovie is used to make a small round hole and a ventricular catheter inserted into the frontal horn. A manometer is used to measure ICP and collect CSF. The dura is now incised longitudinally with the bovie cautery unit. A peel-away introducer can be placed into the frontal horn through each burr hole (Fig. 11). If a single burr hole is used, either the peel-away introducer or the endoscopes cannula-obturator system is used to gain ventricular access. A zero degree scope is inserted and the cyst is localized (Fig. 12). Through the working channel, a YAG laser fiber is inserted or a monopolar or a bipolar unit. The goal of using one of these instruments is to coagulate the cyst's capsule and devascularize it. Typically, once the cyst wall is cauterized and cut, the gelatinous material begins to exit the cyst and spill into the ventricle (Fig. 13). At this point,

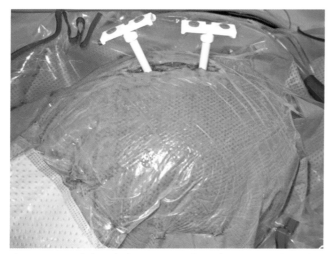

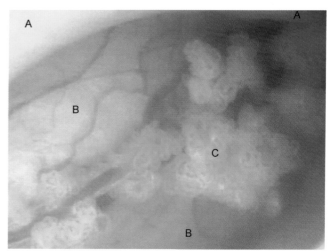

Fig. 11: At each burr hole, a 14-French peel-away introducer has been introduced into the ventricle. An introducer allows access to the endoscope and the other one to a Frazier suction tube.

Fig. 12: Endoscopic view of colloid cyst as seen from the right frontal horn. The columns of the fornix (A) are seen superiorly. The cyst wall (B) filling the foramen of Monro and the choroid plexus (C) are seen at the center of the surgical field.

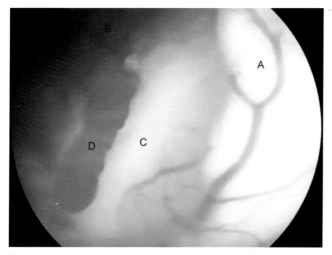

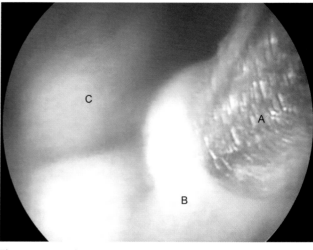

Fig. 13: Endoscopic view of a colloid cyst at the foramen of Monro whose capsular wall has been incised with a YAG laser (B). The column of the fornix (A) devascularized cyst wall (C) and opening into the cyst (D) are visualized.

Fig. 14: Once the cyst wall (C) is incised a gelatinous material is expressed (B) and it can be readily aspirated and removed using a controlled suction instrument (A).

through the second burr hole portal, a controlled suction is inserted and under direct visualization, the contents of the cyst are rapidly and efficiently aspirated (Fig. 14). Once empty, only the cyst wall remains. The suction tip can be used to manipulate the cyst wall by attaching the tip to the wall. Once attached, the laser tip can be used to further fulgurate the cyst and cut its attachments to nearby vascular structures. In order to minimize bleeding, the choroid plexus can be cauterized and devascularized. Further cauterization can be done with the laser or

monopolar units. At this point the majority of the cyst has been removed and the foramina of Monro decompressed (Fig. 15). The ventricles are irrigated with euthermic lactated ringers solution and any bleeding points are cauterized as needed. All the instruments are removed, gelfoam strip is placed at the cortisectomy, and a titanium burr hole cover is placed over the access points. The scalp is closed in standard fashion and the patient is extubated, taken to the recovery room and discharged the following day if asymptomatic and stable.

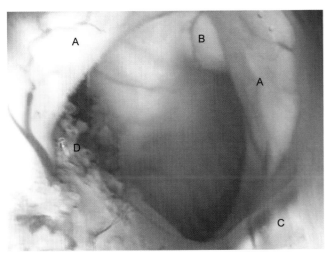

Fig. 15: Following drainage and resection of the colloid cyst, the foramen of Monro is reopened. The columns of the fornix (A) are seen intact and without damage. The anterior commissure of the third ventricle (B) is seen as well as the septal vein (C). The coagulated and devascularized capsule (D) is seen to the left of the image.

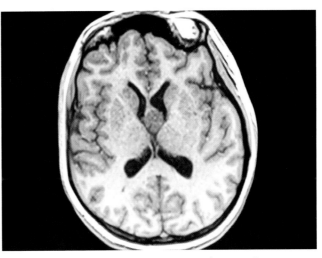

Fig. 16: Case preoperative noncontrasted magnetic resonance imaging depicts colloid cyst of third ventricle.

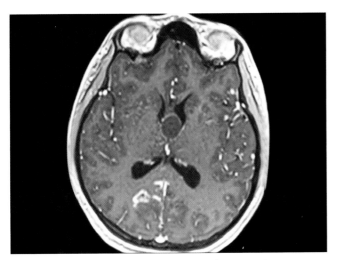

Fig. 17: Case 1 preoperative contrasted magnetic resonance imaging shows colloid cyst at the foramina of Monro.

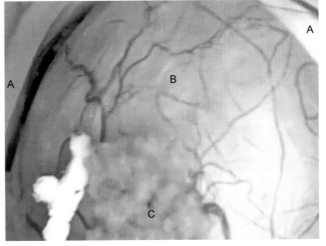

Fig. 18: Case 1 endoscopic view of the patient's colloid cyst column of the right fornix (A), cyst wall (B), and choroid plexus (C), overlying the cyst are seen.

CLINICAL CASES

Case 1

The patient is a 24-year-old right-handed female who presented with a history of chronic headaches (>5 years) which had worsened significantly 3 months prior to admission. She began to experience blurry vision and had several emetic episodes. Her physical exam was normal except for mildly blurred optic disc margins but no papilledema. Diagnostic work up demonstrated a colloid cyst (Figs. 16 and 17). She underwent an uneventful biportal resection of the colloid cyst (Figs. 18 and 19) and was discharged the following day. At a 5-year follow-up, the patient continues to be asymptomatic and without evidence of tumor recurrence (Fig. 20).

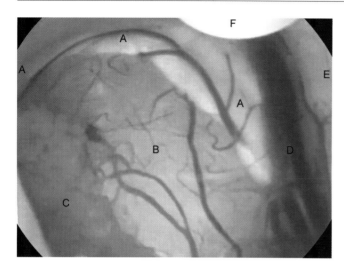

Fig. 19: Case 1 endoscopic view again shows column of the fornix (A), cyst wall (B), choroid plexus (C), septal vein (D), septum pellucidum (E), and peel-away cannula (F) of second portal.

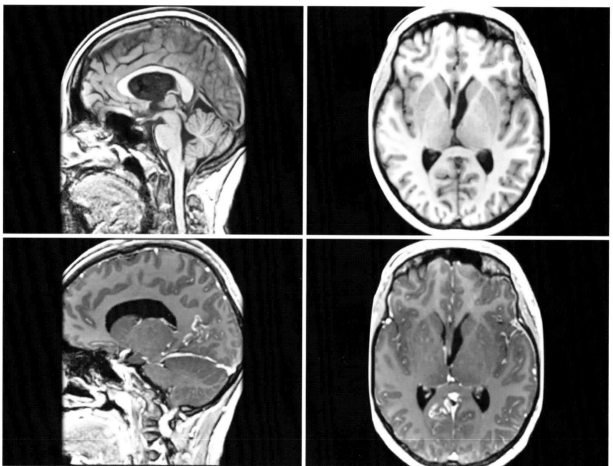

Fig. 20: Case 1 postoperative magnetic resonance imagings contrast and noncontrast 5 years postoperative showing complete cyst resection and no recurrence.[2]

Case 2

The patient is a 41-year-old male who presented with recurring syncopal episodes when bending over and chronic headache, for several years. His neurologic exam was normal. Diagnostic workup demonstrated a colloid cyst (Fig. 21). Surgery was approached via a biportal approach (Fig. 22). He successfully underwent

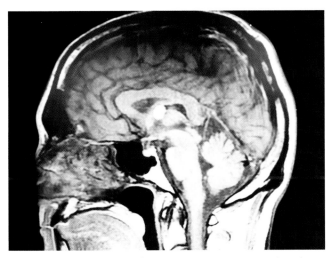

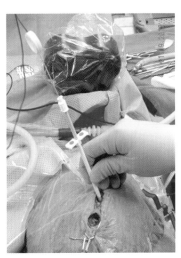

Fig. 21: Case 2 mid-sagittal magnetic resonance imaging shows a hyperintense circular lesion on the anterior roof of the third ventricle consistent with colloid cyst.

Fig. 22: Case 2 surgical photograph shows the peel-away introducer being inserted through the anterior burr hole.

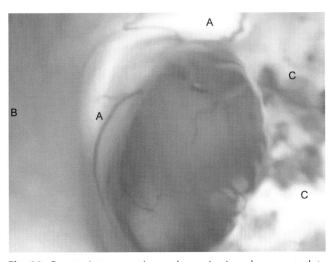

Fig. 23: Case to intraoperative endoscopic view shows complete resection of the cyst. The column of left fornix (A), septum pellucidum (B), and cauterized shrunken capsule (C) are evident.

an endoscopic resection and complete resection of the cyst with opening of the foramen of Monro (Fig. 23). He remains asymptomatic at an 8-year follow-up.

DISCUSSION

Endoscopic management of colloid cysts offers an excellent option for the treating surgeon and for the patient. It can be performed relatively quickly and safely with excellent long-term outcomes. However, it requires that the surgeon has significant endoscopic experience and

it should not be one of the first procedures used by a novice surgeon. While an anterolateral trajectory might be suitable for most subjects, Ibáñez-Botella et al. have recommended using a transventricular transchoroidal approach for patients who have a small foramen of Monro or colloid cysts that protrude minimally into the lateral ventricle.[26] Ravnik et al. reported that they prefer a transcallosal approach because it enables direct surgical access to the cyst area and had the potential to spare the cortex.[6] Chibbaro et al. reported that an anterior transfrontal approach facilitated the reach and removal of cysts exposed from the front; it was especially useful when the cysts were very large and/or located behind the foramen of Monro.[3]

Delitala et al. achieved complete control of cyst wall adhesion to the third ventricle by establishing an entry point 1.5 cm above the supraorbital rim and employing a magnetic neuronavigation tracking system to guide their surgeries.[27] Rangel-Castilla et al. suggested that the optimal entry point for colloid cyst excision is located 42.3 ± 11.7 mm perpendicular to the midline and 46.9 ± 5.7 mm anterior to the coronal suture; however, this location can vary greatly depending on the size of the ventricles.[24] Because of this potential variation, the authors suggested that intraoperative stereotactic navigation be used if available. Failing that, the entry point can be estimated based on the patient's preoperative imaging or, if the patient has ventriculomegaly, an estimated entry point of 4 cm perpendicular to the midline and

4.5 cm anterior to the coronal suture can be used.[24] In the past, the absence of ventriculomegaly was considered by some to be a contraindication to endoscopic resection, but recent studies have concluded that normal-sized ventricles have complication rates that are comparable to the rates of patients with ventriculomegaly.[28] Sribnick et al. reported that patients with or without dilated ventricles presented with similar complaints and similar rates of symptom resolution after endoscopic surgery.[22] Souweidane reported that the success and morbidity rates of endoscopic tumor surgery did not differ between patients in whom hydrocephalus was absent or present.[29] All this evidence suggests that patients who are not hydrocephalic should still be considered viable candidates for endoscopic surgery if they demonstrate common indications for intraventricular biopsy or resection.

CONCLUSION

Endoscopic treatment of colloid cysts is an excellent way for treating these lesions. Although it takes an experienced surgeon, the procedure can be done expeditiously and safely. Outcomes are commensurate with those of open techniques. The surgery is well tolerated. However, care needs to be taken to minimize bleeding and not to cause damage to the ipsilateral column of the fornix. Doing so will lead to loss of short-term memory which may last from several days to several months or longer. Continued vigilance surveillance with MRIs is required to rule out tumor recurrence.

REFERENCES

1. Abdou MS, Cohen AR. Endoscopic treatment of colloid cysts of the third ventricle. Technical note and review of the literature. J Neurosurg. 1998;89(6):1062-8.
2. Boogaarts HD, Decq P, Grotenhuis JA, et al. Long-term results of the neuroendoscopic management of colloid cysts of the third ventricle: a series of 90 cases. Neurosurgery. 2011;68(1):179-87.
3. Chibbaro S, Champeaux C, Poczos P, et al. Anterior transfrontal endoscopic management of colloid cyst: an effective, safe, and elegant way of treatment. Case series and technical note from a multicenter prospective study. Neurosurg Rev. 2014;37(2):235-41.
4. Hernesniemi J, Leivo S. Management outcome in third ventricular colloid cysts in a defined population: a series of 40 patients treated mainly by transcallosal microsurgery. Surg Neurol. 1996;45(1):2-14.
5. Woodley-Cook J, Martinez JL, Kapadia A, et al. Neurosurgical management of a giant colloid cyst with atypical clinical and radiological presentation. J Neurosurg. 2014;121(5):1185-8.
6. Ravnik J, Bunc G, Grcar A, et al. Colloid cysts of the third ventricle exhibit various clinical presentation: a review of three cases. Bosn J Basic Med Sci. 2014;14(3):132-5.
7. Schirmer CM, Heilman CB. Complete endoscopic removal of colloid cyst using a nitinol basket retriever. Neurosurg Focus. 2011;30(4):E8.
8. Azab WA, Salaheddin W, Alsheikh TM, et al. Colloid cysts posterior and anterior to the foramen of Monro: anatomical features and implications for endoscopic excision. Surg Neurol Int. 2014;5:124.
9. Batnitzky S, Sarwar M, Leeds NE, et al. Colloid cysts of the third ventricle. Radiology. 1974;112(2):327-41.
10. Hirano A, Ghatak NR. The fine structure of colloid cysts of the third ventricle. J Neuropathol Exp Neurol. 1974; 33(2):333-41.
11. Little JR, MacCarty CS. Colloid cysts of the third ventricle. J Neurosurg. 1974;40(2):230-5.
12. Kondziolka D, Bilbao JM. An immunohistochemical study of neuroepithelial (colloid) cysts. J Neurosurg. 1989; 71(1):91-7.
13. Macaulay RJ, Felix I, Jay V, et al. Histological and ultrastructural analysis of six colloid cysts in children. Acta Neuropathol. 1997;93(3):271-6.
14. Pollock BE, Huston J 3rd. Natural history of asymptomatic colloid cysts of the third ventricle. J Neurosurg. 1999; 91(3):364-9.
15. de Witt Hamer PC, Verstegen MJ, De Haan RJ, et al. High risk of acute deterioration in patients harboring symptomatic colloid cysts of the third ventricle. J Neurosurg. 2002;96(6):1041-5.
16. Ryder JW, Kleinschmidt-DeMasters BK, Keller TS. Sudden deterioration and death in patients with benign tumors of the third ventricle area. J Neurosurg. 1986;64(2):216-23.
17. Rickert CH, Grabellus F, Varchmin-Schultheiss K, et al. Sudden unexpected death in young adults with chronic hydrocephalus. Int J Legal Med. 2001;114(6):331-7.
18. Desai KI, Nadkarni TD, Muzumdar DP, et al. Surgical management of colloid cyst of the third ventricle—a study of 105 cases. Sur Neurol. 2002;57(5):295-302; discussion 302-4.
19. Mc KW. The surgical treatment of colloid cyst of the third ventricle; a report based upon twenty-one personal cases. Brain. 1951;74(1):1-9.
20. Horn EM, Feiz-Erfan I, Bristol RE, et al. Treatment options for third ventricular colloid cysts: comparison of open microsurgical versus endoscopic resection. Neurosurgery. 2007;60(4):613-8; discussion 8-20.
21. Munich SA, Sazgar M, Grand W, et al. An episode of severely suppressed electrocerebral activity recorded by electroencephalography during endoscopic resection of a colloid cyst. J Neurosurg. 2012;116(2):385-9.
22. Sribnick EA, Dadashev VY, Miller BA, et al. Neuroendoscopic colloid cyst resection: a case cohort with follow-up and patient satisfaction. World Neurosurg. 2014;81(3-4):584-93.
23. Hoffman CE, Savage NJ, Souweidane MM. The significance of cyst remnants after endoscopic colloid cyst

resection: a retrospective clinical case series. Neurosurgery. 2013;73(2):233-7; discussion 7-9.

24. Rangel-Castilla L, Chen F, Choi L, et al. Endoscopic approach to colloid cyst: what is the optimal entry point and trajectory? J Neurosurg. 2014;121(4):790-6.

25. Wilson DA, Fusco DJ, Wait SD, et al. Endoscopic resection of colloid cysts: use of a dual-instrument technique and an anterolateral approach. World Neurosurg. 2013;80(5): 576-83.

26. Ibáñez-Botella G, Dominguez M, Ros B, et al. Endoscopic transchoroidal and transforaminal approaches for resection of third ventricular colloid cysts. Neurosurg Rev. 2014;37(2):227-34; discussion 34.

27. Delitala A, Brunori A, Russo N. Supraorbital endoscopic approach to colloid cysts. Neurosurgery. 2011;69(2 Suppl Operative):ons176-82; discussion ons182-3.

28. Wait SD, Gazzeri R, Wilson DA, et al. Endoscopic colloid cyst resection in the absence of ventriculomegaly.Neurosurgery. 2013;73(1 Suppl Operative):ons39-46;ons46-7.

29. Souweidane MM. Endoscopic surgery for intraventricular brain tumors in patients without hydrocephalus. Neurosurgery. 2005;57(4 Suppl):312-8.

CHAPTER 10

Multiloculated Hydrocephalus

David F Jimenez, David N Garza

INTRODUCTION

Loculated hydrocephalus is a condition in which discrete, fluid-filled compartments form within the ventricular system of the brain.[1] When these compartments become obstructive, cerebrospinal fluid (CSF) accumulates and intracranial pressure increases. This type of hydrocephalus can be described as either uniloculated (in which there is only one obstruction) or multiloculated (in which there are several obstructions). Multiloculated hydrocephalus can arise as a complication of neonatal meningitis, intraventricular hemorrhage, head injury, intracranial surgery, CSF over drainage, shunt infection, and other inflammatory processes.[1-3] The exact pathophysiology behind this condition is still not fully understood. It is thought to involve fibrous adhesion within the ventricles following these inflammatory processes, or it could also be related to the formation of congenital, interventricular, ependymal arachnoid cysts.[4] Salmon first recognized neonatal bacterial meningitis as an etiological factor for multiloculated hydrocephalus in 1970.[3,5] The incidence of bacterial meningitis ranges from 0.13% to 0.37% in full term infants and 1.36% to 2.24% in preterm infants.[6] The incidence of hydrocephalus as a sequela of neonatal meningitis is about 31%.[7] The resultant incidence of hydrocephalus cases caused specifically by neonatal meningitis is fairly uncommon, and the subgroup specifically comprised of multiloculated hydrocephalus cases is rarer still. The scarcity of this patient population within the literature is one of several challenges physicians face when trying to study multiloculated hydrocephalus.

Neonatal bacterial meningitis used to be the most commonly cited etiology for multiloculated hydrocephalus.[8] However, since the mid 80s there have also been a substantial number of reports associating the condition with neonatal intraventricular hemorrhage.[3] Studies published closer to the start of that decade established a clear link between premature infants with low birth weight and intraventricular hemorrhage.[9,10] Subsequent reports estimated that ventriculomegaly occurs in roughly half of that posthemorrhagic population.[11-14] The clear delineation of intraventricular hemorrhage as an independent etiology for multiloculated hydrocephalus was first reported in 1985 by Eller and Pasternak.[3,15]

For both intraventricular hemorrhage and neonatal meningitis, the mechanism responsible for triggering loculation appears to be the initiation of inflammatory pathways caused by ventriculitis.[8,16] Ventriculitis has been associated with 75% to 92% of neonates with meningitis, and chemical ventriculitis is suspected to occur secondary to intraventricular hemorrhage.[3,16,17] A precise pathology explaining how ventriculitis encourages the formation of septations has been explored, but the details have not been fully elucidated. Evidence provided by Schultz and Leeds demonstrated that intraventricular septations are membranes composed of fibroglial elements and polymorphonuclear cells.[18] The authors suggested that these membranes are created by the organization of inflammatory debris or exudate accompanying ventriculitis.[18] The inflammatory response following ventriculitis (which is usually incited by Gram-negative, enteric organisms) stimulates the proliferation of subependymal glial tissue, which leads to the emergence of glial tufts in denuded areas of the ependyma that drive the formation of intraventricular septations.[6,19-21] CSF production and subsequent entrapment within these septations results in cyst expansion. Ventricular septations develop, on average, about 2–4 months following the onset of ventriculitis.[2,3,20] Although the loculations associated with posthemorrhagic cases appear to be triggered by the initiation of the same inflammatory pathways at work in postmeningitic cases, there are some notable differences between the two etiologies.[16] In posthemorrhagic cases, the enlargement of loculations may be related to the severity of hemorrhage.[11,12,15] Within the premature patient population, posthemorrhagic hydrocephalus is often associated with a high incidence of loculation, particularly within the fourth ventricle.[3] In postmeningitic cases, enlargement of the loculated cavities is prompted by the formation of inflammatory exudates; in posthemorrhagic cases, an osmotic gradient created by the lysis of clotted blood likely contributes to any progressive dilation.[3] While additional cyst growth in either population is possible, there is also a chance that the size of a cyst will remain relatively unchanged. This might occur if the lining of the cyst membrane is permeable or infection inhibits the choroid plexus' ability to produce CSF.[20,22]

Mortality rates for multiloculated hydrocephalus have decreased over the years, but the quality of life many patients have is still poor. Ten percent have mild learning disabilities and the rest present with severe cognitive deficits.[23] Clinical features of multiloculated hydrocephalus include headaches, increasing head circumference, a full fontanel, vomiting, seizures, lethargy, hemiparesis, neurological deterioration, developmental delay, and mental retardation.[5,24,25] Predisposing factors include premature birth, low birth weight, perinatal complications, and congenital central nervous system malformations.[23] Typical cases involve infants with meningitis or intraventricular hemorrhage who experience an increase in intracranial pressure that is resistant to shunt treatment. Multiloculated hydrocephalus is characterized as having an evolving disease progression in which the condition worsens with time and necessitates ongoing intervention via surgical procedures of increasing technical difficulty.[16] One challenge that researchers face when discussing any type of loculated hydrocephalus is the ambiguous nomenclature used to classify this condition. Within the literature, loculated hydrocephalus might also be called "septated hydrocephalus" or "complex compartmentalized hydrocephalus"; multiloculated hydrocephalus could refer to a case with a single compartment or multiple compartments; and "ventricular compartmentalization", "ventricular septations", as well as "polycystic", "multicystic", "multiseptae", and "multicompartment"

hydrocephalus have all been used interchangeably to refer to multiloculated hydrocephalus.[1-4,23,26,27] The absence of a consistent naming convention for this condition has hindered the accurate evaluation and comparison of studies that address its diagnosis and treatment.

Andresen and Juhler have taken steps to rectify this problem by proposing new categories for hydrocephalus that address CSF absorption physiology as well as anatomical complexity. Under their classification system, a patient with a single compartment and normal CSF absorption would be designated with *simple uniloculated hydrocephalus* (Fig. 1). If the patient's CSF absorption was abnormal, he or she would be designated with *complex uniloculated hydrocephalus* (Fig. 2). If the patient had two or more compartments, he or she would be described as having one of the following variations of multiloculated hydrocephalus: *physiologically complex multiloculated hydrocephalus* (Fig. 3) (if CSF absorption was abnormal and there were complicating factors), *simple multiloculated hydrocephalus* (if CSF absorption was normal, there were no complicating factors, no anatomical distortion, and few compartments), and *surgically complex multiloculated hydrocephalus* (if CSF absorption was normal and there were no complicating factors, but there was anatomical distortion and/or numerous compartments) (Fig. 4).[1]

Although Andresen and Juhler have taken an important step toward developing a clear, delineated terminology for describing different kinds of loculated hydrocephalus, some authors have expressed skepticism regarding the

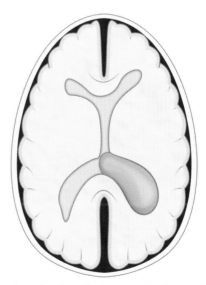

Fig. 1: Simple uniloculated hydrocephalus shows a single separate compartment with normal CSF absorption.

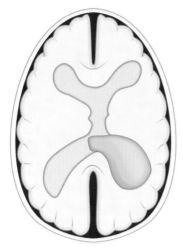

Fig. 2: Complex uniloculated hydrocephalus shows a single compartment with abnormal CSF absorption.

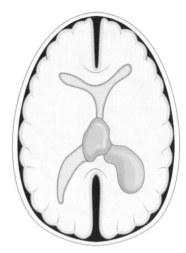

Fig. 3: Simple multiloculated hydrocephalus shows multiple compartments with normal CSF absorption.

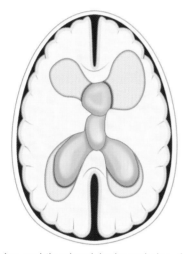

Fig. 4: Complex multiloculated hydrocephalus shows multiple loculated compartments distorted anatomy and abnormal CSF absorption.

implementation of this kind of nomenclature. Akbari et al. believe that such a model would be difficult to apply within a clinical setting, especially because disturbed CSF absorption is a diagnosis of exclusion.[16] They agree that a standardized terminology is needed but believe it would be better for it to exist within a robust, clinically feasible grading model that maintained a high degree of therapeutic efficiency and addressed the variability of this complex condition with an appropriate range of prognoses and treatment options.[16] Because there are a relatively small number of multiloculated hydrocephalus

cases available at any given center, starting a multi-institutional collaborative study might be the best way for researchers to achieve such a goal.

CLINICAL PRESENTATION

While the first case of loculated hydrocephalus was documented by Cushing in 1908, the first case of multi-loculated hydrocephalus was not officially reported until much later, in 1972, by Rhoton and Gomez.[1,28] One of the reasons why multiloculated hydrocephalus used to be so difficult to diagnose was because its symptoms are nonspecific; they can also overlap with other symptoms a patient might be experiencing, like those associated with ventriculitis or regular hydrocephalus. Examples of such symptoms include head enlargement, developmental delay, epilepsy, and hemiparesis.[26] In order to accurately determine whether or not a patient has loculated ventricles, neuroimaging must be used. As the disease progresses, septations often increase in number and vary in thickness; the architecture of the ventricular system appears more obviously distorted, which makes the condition easier to diagnosis using imaging tools.[4] One neuroimaging tool frequently used in the diagnosis of hydrocephalus is computed tomography (CT). It can provide surgeons with the ability to clearly delineate, in a noninvasive manner, ventricular size, web formation, loculation, cyst location, and infarction dimension.[27] However, cyst walls are difficult to visualize on noncontrast CT scans because they are often transparent and have densities that are nearly identical to the density of CSF.[3,4] For this reason, many surgeons consider a contrast-enhanced CT ventriculogram to be the superior preoperative imaging solution.[6] Contrast-enhancement defines the margins of the compartments, visualizes the anatomic relationship between the cavities and normal CSF pathways, and verifies whether or not there is communication with the ventricular system.[25] Before CT was available, multiloculated hydrocephalus was frequently mistaken for shunt malfunction, which resulted in many neurosurgeons performing unnecessary shunt revisions.[3]

Ultrasonography is another helpful imaging option. It is useful in the evaluation of patients with multiloculated ventricles because it can identify the cyst walls, reveal any compartmentalization that has occurred, and provide intraoperative guidance.[6] Schellinger et al. have found ultrasonography to be superior to CT in the identification of intraventricular septations, which appear as solid membranes or firmly interwoven structures.[3] After cyst fenestration has been completed, saline can be injected into the ventricles while a real-time ultrasound is performed in order to verify communication within the ventricular system.[25] Some consider ultrasonography to a superior imaging option because of its noninvasive manner, but the efficacy of its application is greatly dependent on the extent of the operator's experience. Magnetic resonance ventriculography (MRV) is a simple and reliable way to identify obstructive membranes in patients with multiloculated hydrocephalus.[19] It is more sensitive in its ability to detect these septations than a CT scan.[3] Magnetic resonance imaging is capable of providing detailed pictures in three different planes and depicting cyst walls, but its ability to assess CSF flow and determine whether or not there is communication between the compartments of a multiloculated hydrocephalus case is still the subject of debate.[6,19] Although it is more invasive than ultrasonography, it is still safe and practical.

TREATMENT

Although surgical techniques have improved over time, the prognosis for children with multiloculated hydrocephalus is still poor. In the past, some authors considered stereotactic aspiration to be the ideal treatment option because it successfully decompresses the cyst and opens up CSF pathways for uniloculated hydrocephalus cases.[4] However, stereotactic approaches are not capable of completely devascularizing the cyst wall or providing sufficiently wide fenestration.[4,26] For these reasons, they are associated with a high rate of cyst recurrence and cannot be justified in most cases; possible exceptions might include select patients with excessive surgical risk who wish to avoid the morbidity associated with open microsurgery.[25,29]

Open fenestration via microsurgery carries certain risks. Sacrificing bridging veins can result in venous infarction and severe damage can be done to the pericallosal artery, fornices, and subcortical nuclei.[3] Microsurgery has several distinct advantages over other approaches as well. Open fenestration provides excellent visualization of compartments and membranes, a wider and deeper field of view, and better control of bleeding.[23] Because of its overall invasive nature and associated surgical risks, many physicians recommend that open fenestration only be used to treat particularly complicated cases or patients who are refractory to less invasive forms of treatment.[16,23] Multiple shunt placement is the traditional approach to multiloculated hydrocephalus treatment, but it is frequently encumbered by a high rate of complications.[30] Inadequate patient outcomes often necessitate multiple surgical revisions, which can provoke the recurrence of hydrocephalus symptoms. There is also evidence suggesting that each consecutive shunt revision stimulates the formation of new loculations, which diminishes the operative simplicity of any subsequent treatment. With each surgery, the patient's ventricular anatomy grows exponentially more complicated, which forces surgeons to implement treatment strategies of increasing technical difficulty in order to yield the same outcomes.

Shunt-related infection occurs in 5% to 10% of hydrocephalus cases.[2] In the early 90s, Nida et al. and Jamjoom et al. observed that shunt-related infection appeared to incite or hasten the pathology of multiloculated hydrocephalus.[2,8] The mechanism through which this occurs is thought to be similar to the inflammatory pathway discussed earlier involving ventriculitis. Inflammation of the ependyma stimulates the proliferation of subependymal glial tissue, which collects exudate and debris to form fibroglial webs.[2] The physical trauma of shunt implantation can also potentially advance the progression of hydrocephalus. Direct ependymal trauma sustained during catheter insertion might trigger loculations through the formation of fibroglial septa.[3,23] After they are embedded, the ventricular catheters can potentially become a nidus for bacteria that spurs on additional cystic formation through infection.[25] Studies conducted by Oi et al. suggest that the CSF overdrainage via a ventricular shunt

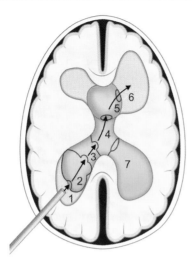

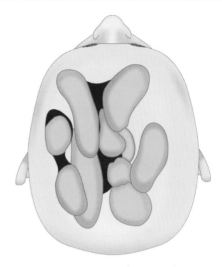

Fig. 5: A patient with complex multiloculated hydrocephalus can be successfully treated with endoscopic techniques which allow all of the separate compartments to be converted into a single, shuntable compartment. In this case, a single occipital-parietal approach is performed. Often times, a biportal approach may be necessary to perform the surgery. (Numbers 1–7 refer to the separate compartments in a case of multiloculated hydrocephalus. The arrows indicate the path taken by the endoscope during the process of fenestrating the compartments).

Fig. 6: Artistic representation of a typical patient with complex multiloculated hydrocephalus showing 11 separate compartments in both lateral ventricles.

system can also isolate ventricular compartments, cause morphological changes in CSF pathways, and alter intracranial pressure dynamics.[31]

There are some authors who speculate that, outside of any infection-related stimulus, the debris of intracranial surgical intervention itself promotes hydrocephalus. Marquardt et al. suggested that proteinic precipitation originating from the surface of a surgical wound washes into the ventricle where it creates arachnoid granulations that inhibit the absorption of CSF.[32] The intraventricular precipitation might also act as a chemical irritant, which can possibly lead to denudation and glial proliferation through the formation of thin septa and the isolation of compartments.[3] If this pathology is accurate, then it means that any type of intracranial surgical intervention carries with it a risk of inciting or perpetuating hydrocephalus symptoms. For this reason, shunting alone may not exclusively be responsible for hydrocephalus recurrence, but there are still other complications endemic to that specific procedure that prevent it from being an ideal, long-term treatment strategy for multiloculated hydrocephalus.

Shunts can malfunction for a variety of reasons, including scarring and cystic collapse around the catheter tip.[25] When previously decompressed compartments collapse

and chronically inflamed ependymal surfaces adhere to each other, new loculations can form.[16] It is possible that these loculations will interfere with ventricular system drainage and cause further shunt malfunction or contribute to recurrent shunt infection.[8,20] As an additional consequence, any local infection will become more difficult to treat as the complexity of compartmentalization increases because loculations impair the diffusion of leukocytes and antibiotics within the ventricular system.[3] All these factors complicate the treatment of multiloculated hydrocephalus and often require a patient to undergo multiple shunt revisions.

Endoscopic cyst fenestration is currently considered by many to be the ideal, initial therapy for multiloculated hydrocephalus.[4,16,25] The procedure works by combining the patient's ventricular compartments into a minimum number and establishing connections to functioning CSF compartments[33] (Fig. 5). The ultimate goal is to reduce the number of proximal shunt catheters and shunt revisions a patient requires or, if possible, avoid shunting altogether[34] (Figs. 6 to 11). Due to a high degree of ventricular complexity or other complicating factors, there are many cases in which endoscopic fenestration is not capable of serving as the exclusive, curative treatment approach to multiloculated hydrocephalus. Under those circumstances, endoscopy can still be used to simplify and stabilize overly-complicated or dysfunctional shunt systems. The outlook for multiloculated hydrocephalus

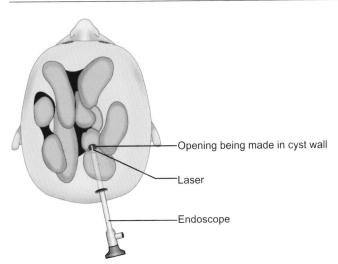

Opening being made in cyst wall

Laser

Endoscope

Fig. 7: The right ventricular system can be endoscopically approached via an occipital portal. Beginning with the cyst closest to the portal, a fenestration is made in order to begin communicating the loculated compartments.

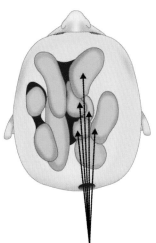

Trajectory used by scope and laser to open and communicate the right side

Fig. 8: Using Image Guidance, the endoscope can be used to sequentially communicate all of the compartments on that side, as seen by the different trajectory arrows.

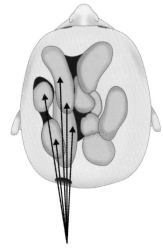

Fig. 9: A similar maneuver can be done on the contralateral side via a separate portal.

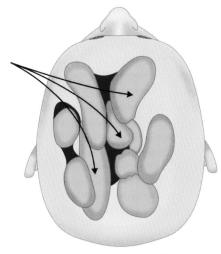

Fig. 10: If during an intraoperative ventriculogram or CT scan, it is demonstrated that residual frontal compartments remain loculated, a third portal can be used to fully communicate all of the compartments.

was traditionally severe, but encouraging results reported by several authors within the literature suggest that neuroendoscopic surgery may help improve its prognosis in the immediate future.[4,16,23]

The first endoscopic fenestration of a ventricular cyst in a child was reported by Kleinhaus et al. in 1982.[6,35] The patient was readmitted for recurrent hydrocephalus and seizures, but the area drained by the shunt remained collapsed after the initial procedure.[35] Several years later, endoscopic approaches to loculated hydro-

cephalus were attempted by Powers in 1986 and Heilman et al. in 1991.[6] Although their studies produced encouraging results, their patient populations were too small to offer conclusive evidence.[26] In 1995, Lewis et al. reported one of the first extensive endoscopic fenestration studies in which the authors operated on 21 patients with uniloculated hydrocephalus and 13 patients with multiloculated hydrocephalus. Endoscopic cyst fenestration reduced the shunt revision rate from 3.04 per year before endoscopy to 0.25 per year after the procedure.[25] In 2003,

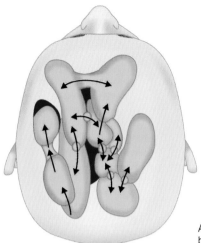

Arrows show connection between all compartments

Fig. 11: At the end of the procedure, all of the different compartments are able to communicate and a single shunt is needed to deal with the remaining communicating hydrocephalus.

Nowoslawska et al. conducted an even larger study of patients who suffered specifically from multiloculated hydrocephalus; 47 were treated endoscopically and 80 were treated using traditional shunting techniques. The authors demonstrated that patients who were treated using neuroendoscopic techniques had better clinical results and fewer complications than those patients who underwent conventional, complicated shunt implantation.[34] Endoscopic techniques decreased the number of operative procedures necessary to complete therapy, made simple shunt implantation possible, and reduced shunt revision rates. The rate of reoperation for the children treated with conventional shunting techniques was 3.949 operations a year; they needed, on average, 7.050 procedures during the duration of their therapy.[34] The rate of reoperation for children treated neuroendoscopically was 1.0232 operations a year; they needed, on average, 1.7660 procedures during the entire duration of their therapy.[34] A study conducted by El-Ghandour in 2008 also determined that endoscopic approaches were associated with better results: lower morbidity and mortality rates as well as shorter recovery times.[26] That same study affirmed Nowoslawska et al.'s observation regarding endoscopy's greater operative simplicity. In El-Ghandour's patient population, shunt revision rates were reduced from 2.9 per year before fenestration to only 0.2 per year after fenestration.[26]

When shunt systems are unavoidable and hindered by a high degree of ventricular compartmentalization, the goal of endoscopic fenestration is to restore communication between the isolated loculations in order to enable a single proximal catheter to drain all the intracranial CSF cavities. Occasionally, it might be necessary for a patient to undergo multiple neuroendoscopic surgeries in order to achieve that ideal outcome. Over the years, in published series, success rates for the management of hydrocephalus using neuroendoscopic approaches and a single shunt have ranged from 61.8% to 100%.[30,34,36] Symptomatic compartmentalizations, the enlargement of an isolated compartment on serial CT scans, shunt failure, and shunt infection should all be considered indications to simplify a multiloculated hydrocephalus patient's preexisting shunt system using a neuroendoscopic approach.[3]

A patient's ventricular complexity and treatment history both play roles in determining the long-term success of endoscopic surgery. In the study conducted by Lewis et al., the authors determined that patients with multiloculated hydrocephalus had a nearly fivefold increased risk (relative risk 4.85) for shunt malfunction and more than a twofold increased risk (relative 2.43) for cyst recurrence when compared to uniloculated hydrocephalus patients.[25] In that same study, patients who had shunt placement prior to undergoing endoscopic cyst fenestration more frequently required additional endoscopic procedures: six out of 12 previously shunted patients (50%) required additional cyst fenestration, whereas only two of 22 patients without previous shunting (9%) required additional cyst fenestration.[25] In a study conducted by El-Ghandour, all uniloculated hydrocephalus patients who had previously undergone shunt treatment required repeated endoscopic cyst fenestration. None of those patients were ever able to become shunt-independent because of the postoperative gliosis induced by previous shunt infection.[37] Because the need for surgical revision is so common within these patient populations, it is recommended that the parents of children with loculated hydrocephalus be made aware of the likelihood of repeat operations as well as the need for close clinical and radiological follow-up.[38]

If a patient's anatomy is distorted because of orientation issues, an endoscopic approach may prove to be problematic because standard navigation techniques become ineffective soon after CSF loss due to brain shift.[33] In an article published by Paraskevopoulos et al., the authors suggest that intraoperative magnetic resonance imaging can be a useful navigation tool to use in conjunction with neuroendoscopy. When combined, these two techniques make orientation easier after brain shift and CSF drainage; they also keep the surgeon aware of membranes that do not have specific intraoperative anatomical landmarks.[33] The potential disadvantages of using intraoperative magnetic resonance (iMR) imaging in conjunction with endoscopy are a prolonged operating time, an increased risk of infection, and the monetary expense.[33] Zuccaro and Ramos employed sonography to achieve real-time image navigation when their patient's anatomy shifted and created confusion.[23]

Flexible endoscopes have been preferred by many authors because of their enhanced maneuverability. However, El-Ghandour et al. opted to use rigid endoscopes in their comprehensive multiloculated hydrocephalus patient studies. They asserted that rigid endoscopes have greater light intensity and superior optics that provide better visualization. Their limited maneuverability can be offset by carefully selecting the burr hole placement site and widening the outer edge of the burr hole in order to allow more movement and permit different trajectories.[26] El-Ghandour, Zuccaro, and Ramos all believe that it is beneficial to make the fenestration very wide, at least 1 cm or more in diameter, in order to offset the high incidence of reclosure caused by the low pressure differential across cyst walls as well as the inflammatory nature of this condition.[23,26] It is critical that the surgeon takes care to enlarge the fenestration with forceps, scissors, or a Fogarty balloon and devascularize the septa in order to inhibit any potential regrowth.[23]

CLINICAL CASE 1

The patient is a 7-month-old child who was born with spina bifida and ventriculomegaly. On his second day of life he underwent a successful closure of his lumbosacral myelomeningocele. A ventriculoperitoneal shunt was placed for progressive macrocrania. Three weeks after the shunt, he returned with failure to thrive, fevers, somnolence, and decreased feedings. A diagnostic work up with CT scan showed progressive enlargement of the ventricles with suspicion of multiloculation. A ventriculogram was done with intrathecal contrast which revealed a total of 11 separate cysts (Figs. 12 and 13).

A decision was made to take the patient to surgery to perform an endoscopic fenestration of the separate intraventricular compartments. Given the complexity of the anatomy, preoperative scans were loaded into the Brainlab image guided station and the patient was appropriately registered (Fig. 14). As is the case with these complex and longer cases, a sitting stool with arm rests (Fig. 15) was utilized. A YAG laser inserted through a flexible endoscope was used to devascularize and create

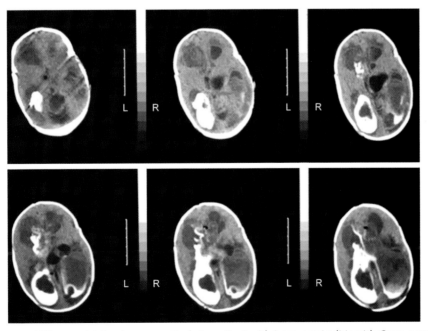

Fig. 12: Intrathecal contrasted CT scan obtained preoperatively in patient with intraventriculitis with Gram-negative organisms, fevers, somnolence, and poor feeding.

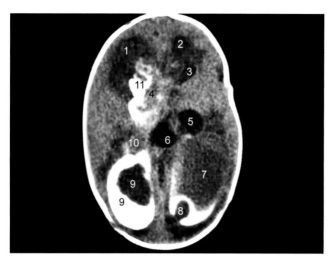

Fig. 13: Axial preoperative CT scan shows a multicompartmental picture with at least 11 differently isolated and noncommunicating compartments.

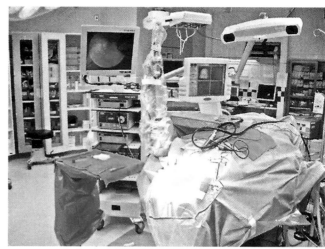

Fig. 14: Operating room set-up using image guidance to perform the complex task of communicating all compartments with endoscopic assistance.

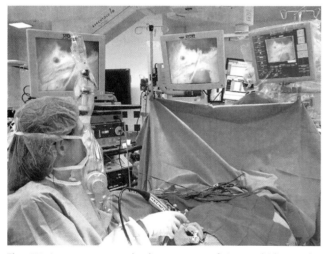

Fig. 15: Long cases can lead to surgeon fatigue which can be successfully minimized by using an operating stool with arm rests. This allows for arm/elbow/hand stabilization and support.

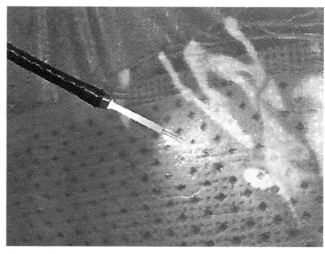

Fig. 16: These cases can be safely and ideally done using a laser. TAG or KTP lasers can be used through the working channel of a flexible endoscopy, as seen on this photo. The red light is an aiming beam.

the fenestrations (Fig. 16). A 14-French peel-away introducer was used to enter the ventricle via a right sided occipital approach. Upon entrance, a thick membrane was encountered which was fenestrated with the YAG laser (Fig. 17). Multiple compartments were entered sequentially (Figs. 18 and 19). A Gram stain obtained during surgery revealed a Gram-negative rod which grew *Enterobacter cloaca*. Once the right ventricular system was felt to be decompartmentalized, an intraoperative CT ventriculogram was done (Fig. 20) which demonstrated

successful fenestration and dye dissemination throughout that ventricle. The procedure continued and the contralateral side was similarly fenestrated and both right and left systems communicated. A postoperative CT scan corroborated the findings (Fig. 21). A single left frontal external ventricular drain was left in place and patient was treated successfully with both intravenous and intrathecal antibiotics. Subsequently, a right frontal VP shunt was placed and the patient was discharged in stable condition.

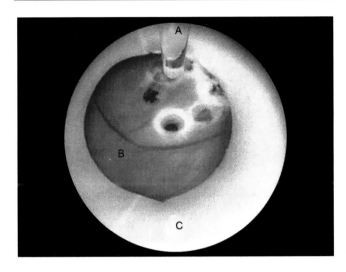

Fig. 17: A 14-French peel-away introducer (C) has been used to access the ventricle. This image shows the laser probe (A) and the multiple small openings being made on the cyst wall (B). These openings are made circumferentially and then connected.

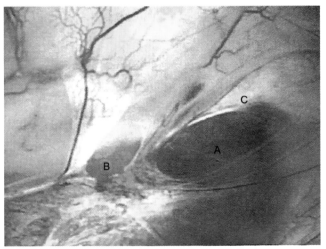

Fig. 18: Endoscopic view of right lateral ventricle showing the fornix (C) and choroid plexus (B). A membrane (A) is seen covering the expanded foramen of Monro.

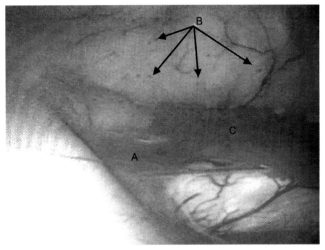

Fig. 19: A view toward the occipital horn/trigone shows a membrane covering the occipital horn (A) the choroid plexus (C) is seen as well as multiple hyper pigmented areas on the ventricular walls (B) indicating the presence of an infection.

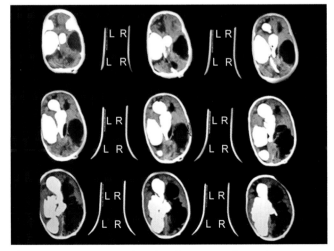

Fig. 20: An intraoperative, intrathecally contrasted scan shows successful fenestration and communication of the right ventricular system.

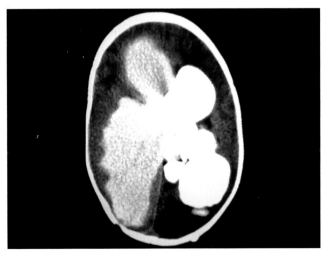

Fig. 21: Postoperative CT scan with intrathecal contrast shows complete fenestration of both ventricular system in same patient.

CLINICAL CASE 2

A twenty-five-month-old female presented with nausea, vomiting, poor appetite and headaches. Neurologic examination was normal except for blurred optic disc margins. MRIs were obtained which demonstrated a case of simple uniloculated hydrocephalus, with a large cyst located in the left atrium of the lateral ventricle causing mass effect (Figs. 22 to 24). A decision was made to treat with endoscopic fenestration of the cyst. Image guidance during surgery was crucial to obtaining a successful result (Fig. 25). The patient underwent an uneventful and successful fenestration of the cyst into the lateral ventricle via an occipital approach. The symptoms resolved and a postoperative MRI a year later showed a decompressed cyst and normal ventricular size and function (Figs. 26 to 28).

CONCLUSION

A history of intracranial surgical intervention, especially previous shunt placement, tends to predict poor long-term patient outcomes for multiloculated hydrocephalus. These procedures often provoke the recurrence of hydrocephalus by inciting new loculation through the

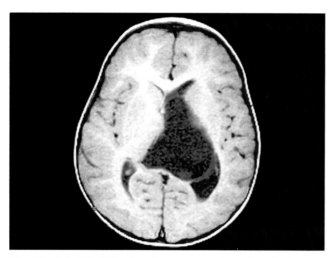

Fig. 22: Axial T1 MRI of patient presented as Case 2 shows a large uniloculated left lateral ventricle with mass effect on the splenium of the corpus callosum and surrounding structures.

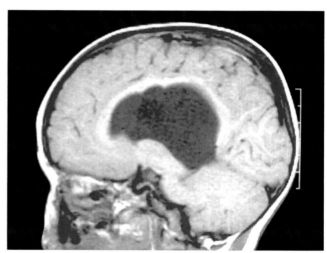

Fig. 23: Sagittal T1 MRI demonstrated elevation and mass effect of the cyst on the body of the corpus callosum.

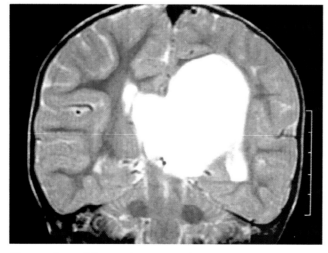

Fig. 24: Coronal T2 MRI depicts very large cyst with compression of surrounding brain.

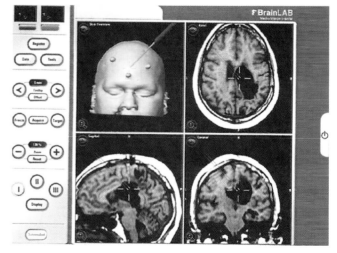

Fig. 25: Screen shot of image guidance with the Brain Lab system used in preparation for fenestration of the cyst.

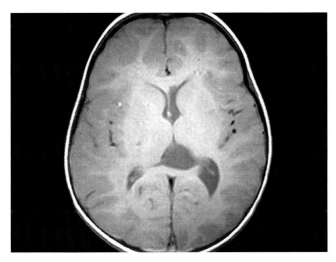

Fig. 26: Axial T1 MRI, one year postoperative demonstrates persistent decompression of the cyst.

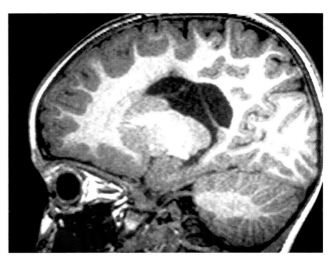

Fig. 27: T1 sagittal post MRI shows collapsed walls of the cyst and no mass effect.

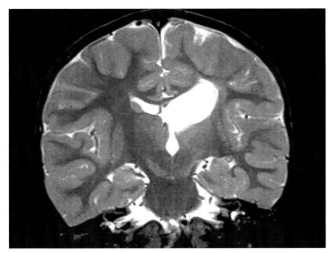

Fig. 28: Coronal T2 MRI a year later after endoscopic cyst fenestration.

inflammatory pathways associated with ventriculitis. Endoscopic cyst fenestration is the ideal initial treatment for multiloculated hydrocephalus due to its minimally invasive nature. Even when it cannot serve as the exclusive curative procedure, it is still capable of simplifying complicated shunt systems and reducing shunt revision rates. Other approaches are worth considering depending on a patient's anatomical features and the degree of their ventricular complexity. Patients who are refractory to endoscopic treatment might be viable candidates for more invasive approaches, such as open fenestration via craniotomy.

REFERENCES

1. Andresen M, Juhler M. Multiloculated hydrocephalus: a review of current problems in classification and treatment. Child's Nerv Syst. 2012;28(3):357-62.
2. Jamjoom AB, Mohammed AA, Al-Boukai A, et al. Multiloculated hydrocephalus related to cerebrospinal fluid shunt infection. Acta Neurochir (Wien). 1996;138(6):714-9.
3. Spennato P, Cinalli G, Carannante G, et al. Multiloculated hydrocephalus. In: Cinalli G, Sainte-Rose C, Maixner W (Eds). Pediatric Hydrocephalus. Milan: Springer; 2005. pp. 219-44.
4. Eshra MA. Endoscopic management of septated, multiloculated hydrocephalus. Alexandria J Med. 2014;50(2):123-6.
5. Salmon JH. Isolated unilateral hydrocephalus following ventriculoatrial shunt. J Neurosurg. 1970;32(2):219-26.
6. Abtin K, Walker M. Endoscopic management of complex hydrocephalus. In: Jimenez D (Ed). Intracranial Endoscopic Neurosurgery. Neurosurgical Topics. Park Ridge, IL: American Association of Neurological Surgeons; 1998.
7. Lorber J, Pickering D. Incidence and treatment of post-meningitic hydrocephalus in the newborn. Arch Dis Child. 1966;41(215):44-50.
8. Nida TY, Haines SJ. Multiloculated hydrocephalus: craniotomy and fenestration of intraventricular septations. J Neurosurg. 1993;78(1):70-6.
9. Ahmann PA, Lazzara A, Dykes FD, et al. Intraventricular hemorrhage in the high-risk preterm infant: incidence and outcome. Ann Neurol. 1980;7(2):118-24.
10. Papile LA, Burstein J, Burstein R, et al. Incidence and evolution of subependymal and intraventricular hemorrhage: a study of infants with birth weights less than 1,500 gm. J Pediatr. 1978;92(4):529-34.

11. Allan WC, Holt PJ, Sawyer LR, et al. Ventricular dilation after neonatal periventricular-intraventricular hemorrhage. Natural history and therapeutic implications. Am J Dis Child. 1982;136(7):589-93.

12. Hill A, Volpe JJ. Normal pressure hydrocephalus in the newborn. Pediatrics. 1981;68(5):623-9.

13. Levene MI, Starte DR. A longitudinal study of post-haemorrhagic ventricular dilatation in the newborn. Arch Dis Child. 1981;56(12):905-10.

14. Ment LR, Duncan CC, Scott DT, et al. Posthemorrhagic hydrocephalus. Low incidence in very low birth weight neonates with intraventricular hemorrhage. J Neurosurg. 1984;60(2):343-7.

15. Eller TW, Pasternak JF. Isolated ventricles following intraventricular hemorrhage. J Neurosurg. 1985;62(3):357-62.

16. Akbari SH, Holekamp TF, Murphy TM, et al. Surgical management of complex multiloculated hydrocephalus in infants and children. Child's Nerv Syst. 2015;31(2):243-9.

17. Berman PH, Banker BQ. Neonatal meningitis. A clinical and pathological study of 29 cases. Pediatrics. 1966;38(1): 6-24.

18. Schultz P, Leeds NE. Intraventricular septations complicating neonatal meningitis. J Neurosurg. 1973;38(5):620-6.

19. Gandhoke GS, Frassanito P, Chandra N, et al. Role of magnetic resonance ventriculography in multiloculated hydrocephalus. J Neurosurg Pediatr. 2013;11(6):697-703.

20. Kalsbeck JE, DeSousa AL, Kleiman MB, et al. Compartmentalization of the cerebral ventricles as a sequela of neonatal meningitis. J Neurosurg. 1980;52(4):547-52.

21. Sandberg DI, McComb JG, Krieger MD. Craniotomy for fenestration of multiloculated hydrocephalus in pediatric patients. Neurosurgery. 2005;57(1 Suppl):100-6.

22. Breeze RE, McComb JG, Hyman S, et al. CSF production in acute ventriculitis. J Neurosurg. 1989;70(4):619-22.

23. Zuccaro G, Ramos JG. Multiloculated hydrocephalus. Child's Nerv Syst. 2011;27(10):1609-19.

24. Albanese V, Tomasello F, Sampaolo S, et al. Neuroradiological findings in multiloculated hydrocephalus. Acta Neurochirurgica. 1982;60(3-4):297-311.

25. Lewis AI, Keiper GL Jr, Crone KR. Endoscopic treatment of loculated hydrocephalus. J Neurosurg. 1995;82(5):780-5.

26. El-Ghandour NM. Endoscopic cyst fenestration in the treatment of multiloculated hydrocephalus in children. J Neurosurg Pediatr. 2008;1(3):217-22.

27. Brown LW, Zimmerman RA, Bilaniuk LT. Polycystic brain disease complicating neonatal meningitis: documentation of evolution by computed tomography. J Pediatr. 1979; 94(5):757-9.

28. Rhoton AL Jr, Gomez MR. Conversion of multilocular hydrocephalus to unilocular. Case report. J Neurosurg. 1972;36(3):348-50.

29. Mathiesen T, Grane P, Lindquist C, et al. High recurrence rate following aspiration of colloid cysts in the third ventricle. J Neurosurg. 1993;78(5):748-52.

30. Spennato P, Cinalli G, Ruggiero C, et al. Neuroendoscopic treatment of multiloculated hydrocephalus in children. J Neurosurg. 2007;106(1 Suppl):29-35.

31. Oi S, Hidaka M, Honda Y, et al. Neuroendoscopic surgery for specific forms of hydrocephalus. Child's Nerv Syst. 1999;15(1):56-68.

32. Marquardt G, Setzer M, Lang J, et al. Delayed hydrocephalus after resection of supratentorial malignant gliomas. Acta Neurochir. 2002;144(3):227-31.

33. Paraskevopoulos D, Biyani N, Constantini S, et al. Combined intraoperative magnetic resonance imaging and navigated neuroendoscopy in children with multicompartmental hydrocephalus and complex cysts: a feasibility study. J Neurosurg Pediatr. 2011;8(3):279-88.

34. Nowoslawska E, Polis L, Kaniewska D, et al. Effectiveness of neuroendoscopic procedures in the treatment of complex compartmentalized hydrocephalus in children. Child's Nerv Syst. 2003;19(9):659-65.

35. Kleinhaus S, Germann R, Sheran M, et al. A role for endoscopy in the placement of ventriculoperitoneal shunts. Surg Neurol. 1982;18(3):179-80.

36. Heilman CB, Cohen AR. Endoscopic ventricular fenestration using a "saline torch". J Neurosurg. 1991;74(2):224-9.

37. El-Ghandour NM. Endoscopic cyst fenestration in the treatment of uniloculated hydrocephalus in children. J Neurosurg Pediatr. 2013;11(4):402-9.

38. Schulz M, Bohner G, Knaus H, et al. Navigated endoscopic surgery for multiloculated hydrocephalus in children. J Neurosurg Pediatr. 2010;5(5):434-42.

CHAPTER 11

Endoscopic Neuronavigation and Image Guidance

David F Jimenez, Colin T Son

INTRODUCTION

Stereotaxy and image guidance have been combined with neuroendoscopy since the widespread adaptation of frame-based stereotactic systems in clinical practice.[1] The eventual ubiquity of computer tomography greatly improved the accuracy of frame-based stereotactic neurosurgery.[2,3] The utility of image guidance during neuroendoscopy has been further advanced with improvements in magnetic resonance imaging (MRI). In 1991 Hayakawa et al. described the first clinical use of a frameless stereotactic system with real time intraoperative image guidance and other systems quickly followed.[4-6] These systems were quickly adapted for use during neuroendoscopy.[7-10]

Nowadays, intraoperative image guidance is widely used during neuroendoscopy and is an imperative tool for the neurosurgeon undertaking such procedures to understand.

PRINCIPLES OF INTRAOPERATIVE IMAGE-GUIDED NAVIGATION

Frameless intraoperative image guidance systems have been developed from a number of principles. Today, two major types of systems remain in widespread use: (1) optical image guidance systems and (2) electromagnetic image guidance systems. The former uses a camera to detect the reflection or transmission of infrared light off special attachments to operative instruments. The latter senses the strength of an electromagnetic field produced by special attachments to operative instruments. Many, but not all, optical systems require rigid fixation of the patient following registration. The camera must see the patient in the same position relative to the patient reference array throughout the course of the procedure. Systems based on the detection of electromagnetic fields allow for movement of the patient's head intraoperatively as the reference point is generally affixed to the patient. These systems also remove the line of sight limitation inherent to camera-based systems. These units localize a patient in three-dimensions (3D) and compare to preoperative computed tomographic and/or MRI following registration. The surgical tools and instruments are then identified in relation to their location to the patient. Recent advances allow nonfiducial-based surface registration of patients to couple to their preoperative imaging as well as the integration of intraoperatively obtained images.

TECHNICAL DETAILS OF INTRAOPERATIVE IMAGE-GUIDED NAVIGATION IN NEUROENDOSCOPY

There are many particular commercially available surgical navigation systems in use and a description of all of them is beyond the scope of this chapter. Discussed herein are the basic steps in the utilization of image-guided navigation during neuroendoscopy and the specifics of three systems in widespread use: (1) Kick/Curve (Brainlab, Munich, Germany), (2) StealthStation (Medtronic, Dublin, Ireland) and (3) Nav3/Nav3i (Stryker, Kalamazoo, Michigan, USA). Frameless real-time image navigation starts with preoperative obtainment of high-quality volumetric computed tomography (CT) and/or MRI. All three systems allow the importation of the no-gantry, thin slice images (typically < 3 mm) via CD/DVD-ROM, wired or wireless connection to a picture archiving and communication system (PACS) or USB flash drive. Various image modalities and series can be merged and

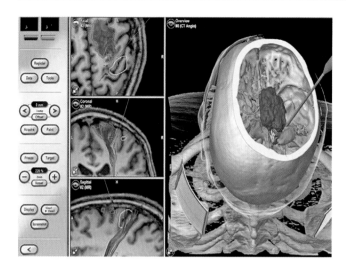

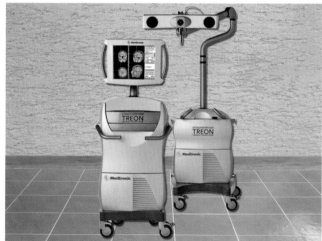

Fig. 1: Preoperative MRI and CT angio data have been entered into a Brainlab workstation for preoperative planning. The data can be manipulated to demonstrate the primary pathology (tumor) as well as the pathways of white matter tracks (tractography) to aid the surgeon with safe lesion resection. (MRI: Magnetic resonance imaging; CT: Computed tomography).
Courtesy: Brainlab.

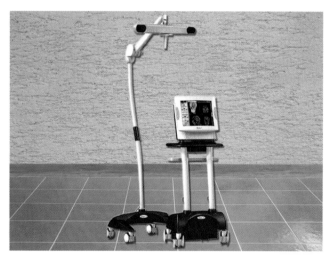

Fig. 2: Image of one of the Brainlab stations used for neuro-navigation. On the left, the tower with the adjustable sensor cameras is seen. On the right, the workstation is seen. These are mobile units that can be moved around the operating room as needed.
Courtesy: Brainlab.

Fig. 3: Medtronic's TREON StealthStation imports images from various sources (X-ray, CT, MRI) and reconstructs 3D images which can be manipulated as needed for intraoperative navigation. Can be used in brain, spine and ear, and nose and throat procedures. (CT: Computed tomography; MRI: Magnetic resonance imaging).
Courtesy: Medtronic.

manipulated prior to registration to allow for this data to be viewed and used during intraoperative navigation (Fig. 1). This may be particularly useful in cases of endoscopy of the skull base, where CT may delineate the bony features on approach and various MRI series may show the intracranial pathology and vascular structures.

The importation, fusion and preregistration manipulation of the image data not only differs between systems but involves user interfaces and capabilities which are constantly being improved upon by manufacturers. Therefore, effective use of any image guidance systems requires the continuing education and hands-on experience of the neuroendoscopist. In general, the initial step in the

Brainlab or Medtronic (Figs. 2 and 3) systems involves the selection of the tracking method (optical or electromagnetic) to be used. The procedure begins with the importation of the images via CD/DVD-ROM, PACS or USB into the workstation. Volumetric image series are selected as the primary images from which the computer will build a 3D model for adequate navigation. Following this, other image series, including nonvolumetric sequences, can be fused with the primary volumetric series. For instance a surgeon doing an endoscopic transsphenoidal resection of a pituitary adenoma may use a CT scan to build the 3D

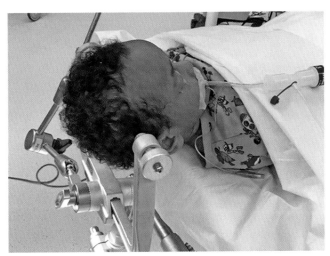

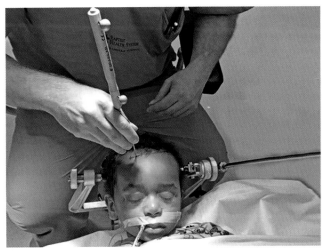

Fig. 4: A 3-year-old male with a complex intraventricular cyst has been placed on a three point rigid Mayfield cranial fixation clamp. To the left of the patient's head is a standard cranial reference array with three marker spheres that track the location of the patient's head.

Fig. 5: The surgeon uses a wireless soft-touch pointer for registration, surface matching, and verification of anatomical surface landmarks. Eliminates the need for registration rescans and thus reduces radiation exposure.

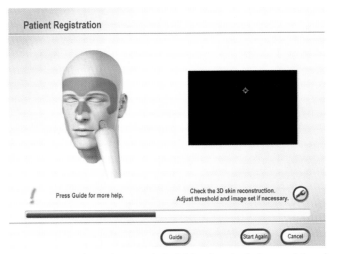

Fig. 6: Screenshot of patient's facial landmarks being registered with hand-held laser tracker and area being registered (green area).

model of the patient but then fuse it to a T2 weighted MRI sequence. This fusion allows for tracking within the MRI images so that intraoperatively, the surgeon can navigate either based on the CT or the MRI scans and switch between them. As with most image viewing software, the images can now be manipulated for brightness and contrast. Further preregistration planning may be done, so as to "paint" and highlight the pathology or to plan trajectories with the marking of both entry and end points.

Registration and navigation with the optical tracking options of the Brainlab Kick/Curve and Medtronic

StealthStation systems require initial patient fixation in a Mayfield head holder (Fig. 4). Both systems use an infrared light emitter and camera distant from the patient to track the reflection of the infrared light from attachments to instruments in relation to a fixed patient reference array. In both systems the patient reference array attaches directly to the head holder prior to registration. Non-fiducial registration involves the identification of surface points on the patient with a wired or wireless tracer (Fig. 5) or, in the case of the Brainlab systems, the option for a laser tracing of surface landmarks (Fig. 6). The system camera should be positioned in such a way to view both the patient reference array and tracker constantly during patient registration (Fig. 7). The nonsterile patient reference array used for registration is then removed and, following patient prepping and draping, replaced by a sterile array through the drapes. Landmark registration follows (Figs. 8 to 10). Following registration, time should be taken to select the views of the navigation which will be most helpful to the surgeon. Some systems allow up to six simultaneous views on the screen at once. Options include, but are not limited to, axial, coronal, sagittal, oblique and in line views from the tip of the navigated instrument.

Once registration is complete and the views have been set up to the surgeon's liking, these systems can aid in the incision and burr hole placement planning with provided pointers and stylets. Offsets can be placed on the tips of the stylets by the computer to measure distance and plan intracranial trajectories prior to incision. In addition, for

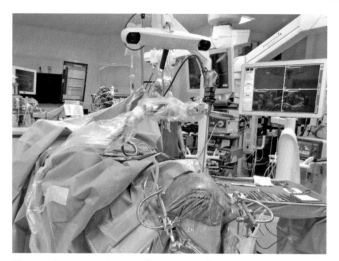

Fig. 7: Intraoperative sterile set-up of an endoscopic neuro-navigation case. The rigid endoscope has been set on a pneumatic Mitaka holder. The infrared sensor/camera has been placed above the patient and coupled with a reference array. The monitor is placed as such that the surgeon can easily visualize the instruments and endoscope movements inside the patient's brain.

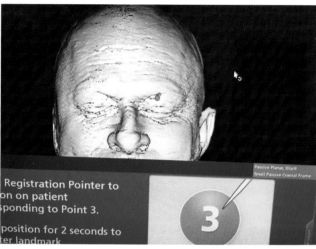

Fig. 8: Screenshot of the navigation station prompting the surgeon to register the wireless pointer to the patient's left mid-supraorbital point.

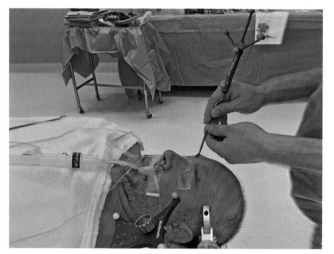

Fig. 9: The surgeon registers the wireless pointer to the patient's left supraorbital midpoint as prompted.

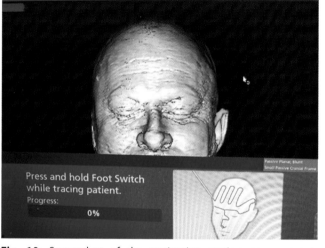

Fig. 10: Screenshot of the navigation station now prompts the surgeon to continuously landmark surface of the face and forehead as seen on the right lower diagram.

intraoperative guidance, both systems have a variety of reference arcs for attachment to virtually any rigid surgical instrument for their real time tracking within the surgical field (Fig. 11). On an endoscope, reference arcs should traditionally be attached to the irrigation ports to avoid occlusion of the working port or to the body of the scope (Fig. 12). The endoscope requires registration prior to accurate tracking by the optical system. Registration is straightforward for both systems requiring the identification of the endoscope length and diameter by placement of the end of the endoscope within the appropriate diameter reference in the provided sterile calibration device once the reference arc has been attached. This allows the systems to know the length of the endoscope, essentially the distance from where the reference arc is attached to the tip and allows the real time tracking of the endoscope tip intracranially as long as the reference arc is visible to the camera (Figs. 13 to 16). Brainlab uses a different system for endoscope registration, the instrument calibration matrix (Fig. 17).

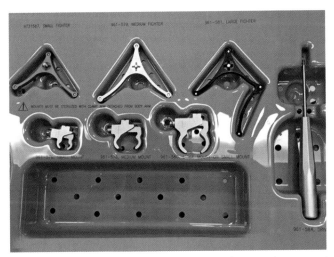

Fig. 11: A tray showing the various attachment clamps and reference arrays that can be attached to any instrument, including endoscopes. Once attached to the instrument, it can be registered with the system and adequately tracked.

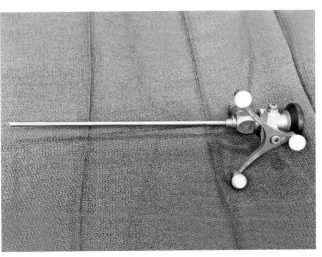

Fig. 12: Photograph shows a rigid 4-mm endoscope with a reference array (orange instrument) and marking spheres attached to the body of the endoscope with a rigid clamp.

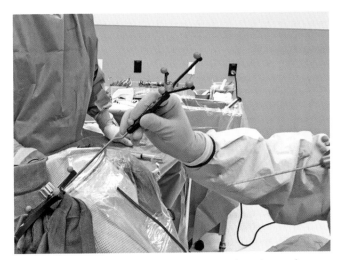

Fig. 13: The surgeon's first step in registering the endoscope includes registering the pointer to the standard cranial reference array which is attached to the Mayfield clamp.

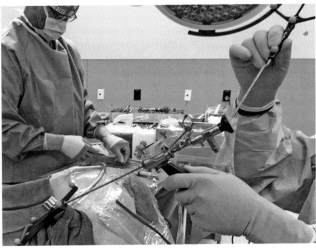

Fig. 14: The surgeon registers the tip of the endoscope to the cranial reference array and the pointer to the back of the endoscope in direct line to the tip of the scope.

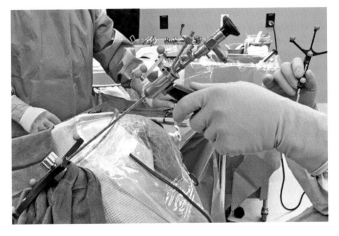

Fig. 15: Finally, the tip of the endoscope is registered to the cranial reference array. The tip of the endoscope can be tracked inside the patient's brain.

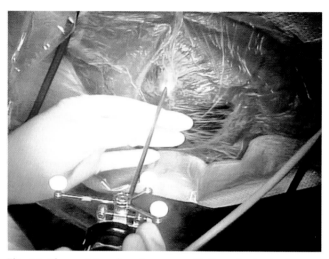

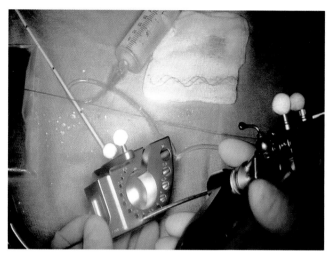

Fig. 16: The registered endoscope, with the attached reference array and marking spheres being introduced into the patient's brain.

Fig. 17: Brainlab's instrument calibration matrix (in the surgeon's left hand) has different size holder into which to place different size endoscopes or instruments. The rigid endoscope is inserted into the proper size hole along with its attached tracker. Both instruments are then registered to the system's sensing camera above the patient.

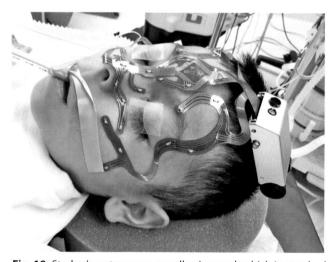

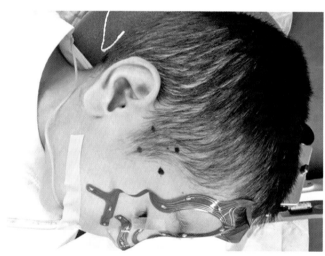

Fig. 18: Stryker's system uses an adhesive mask which is attached to the patient's forehead, cheeks, and nose with markers which are registered automatically by the navigation station.

Fig. 19: Stryker's mask on patient's face, side view demonstrates the area where the temporal arachnoid cyst comes closest to the surface (block dots). The proper entry port has been selected for this patient who presented with a large, symptomatic right middle fossa arachnoid cyst.

The Stryker Nav3/Nav3i system is a wholly optical tracking system with many similarities to the optical tracking options discussed above. Notable differences include the ability to navigate without rigid fixation via a post kit mounted to the skull through a small incision and the ability for automatic mask registration of the patient. In the more traditional method of use the patient's head is again fixed within a Mayfield head holder. For automatic registration, a provided mask is attached to the patient's face via underlying adhesive (Figs. 18 and 19). The mask covers the bridge of the nose, forehead, and brow. LEDs within the mask are visible to the camera. The Communication Unit is attached to the mask and automatic registration initiated by holding the select button on the Communication Unit. The patient reference array, referred to as a Universal Tracker within Stryker nomenclature, is then attached to the Mayfield and made visible to the camera. The position of the LEDs on the patient's mask is compared by the software to the fixed position of the Universal Tracker to complete registration. In light of the attachment of the Universal Tracker to the fixed Mayfield a minimally invasive skull post may be screwed to the skull via a small incision prior to final prepping and draping. In this case the fixation of the reference point to the patient allows for head movement and repositioning intraoperatively without disruption of navigation. In similar fashion to other optical systems, the endoscope must be attached to a tracker and its length and diameter registered prior to navigation in the provided calibration unit.

Rigid fixation of the head during neurosurgery is at times not ideal, including during some neuroendoscopic procedures. The need for neuronavigation without fixation within a Mayfield head holder has been solved for optical tracking systems by the surgical fixation of a reference point to the patient's skull and for electromagnetic tracking systems by the fixation of a reference point to the skin[11] (Fig. 20). The ability to noninvasively track patients out of rigid fixation is seen by some as a major benefit of electromagnetic image guidance systems. In addition electromagnetic systems solve the problem of line of sight inherent to optical systems. In optical systems infrared LEDs or infrared reflections must be visible

to a camera and the position of the surgeon or patient in relation to the surgical instrument or reference array may hamper visibility and thus navigation.[12] Today electromagnetic systems have accuracy similar to optical systems.[12] One significant limitation of electromagnetic systems is metallic interference. This has been improved greatly upon in recent iterations of these systems but continues to limit navigable surgical instruments to those specially designed.[13] As such neither Brainlab's Kick EM or Medtronic's StealthStation AxiEM easily allow for the real time tracking of the endoscope position itself.

Use of the Brainlab and Medtronic electromagnetic systems commences very similarly to their optical tracking counterpart. Following the loading of the preoperatively obtained volumetric imaging into the computer, the patient is positioned in reference to the tracking unit which in both systems fits in an arm which attaches to the operating bed railing. The connection panel interfaces between the tracking unit, the patient reference, all navigation tools, and the navigation system. The patient reference in both systems is a marker which affixes to the forehead via adhesive. Once the patient reference has been affixed to the patient's forehead and the patient reference, tracking unit, and registration stylet attached to the connection panel surface registration continues similarly to the procedure for Brainlab and Medtronic's optical tracking solutions with the notation that only stylet registration, and not touchless laser registration, is possible with the electromagnetic systems. Provided pointers and stylets attach to the connection panel and navigate in real time. As in the optical tracking options, they allow for both pre-incision planning and intraoperative identification of position. In addition, both manufacturers offer specialized suction units which after being calibrated will track in real time as well.

While no review has definitively demonstrated such conclusion, the use of intraoperative image-guided navigation during neuroendoscopy has been posited to reduce complications and improve outcomes.[14,15] The major applications for this technology continue to grow. Initially limited to pre-incision planning, currently the ability to easily and accurately track the rigid endoscope, as well as the widespread adaptation of electromagnetic technology has greatly expanded the role for navigation during neuroendoscopy (Fig. 21). Intraoperative image-guided navigation has been demonstrated in the literature as particularly useful in cases intra- or

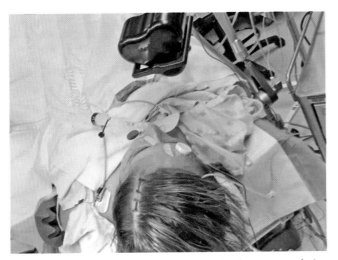

Fig. 20: Medtronic's electromagnetic navigation system being used for a patient with a colloid cyst. The reference magnet is placed on a holder near and in front of the patient's head.

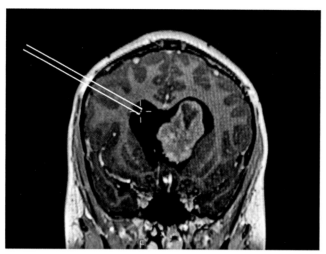

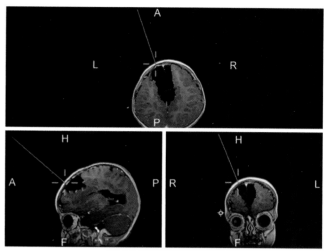

Fig. 21: Once registered the tip of the endoscope is seen entering the patient's right frontal horn.

Fig. 22: Intraoperative navigation in the fenestration of a symptomatic and enlarging midline arachnoid cyst.

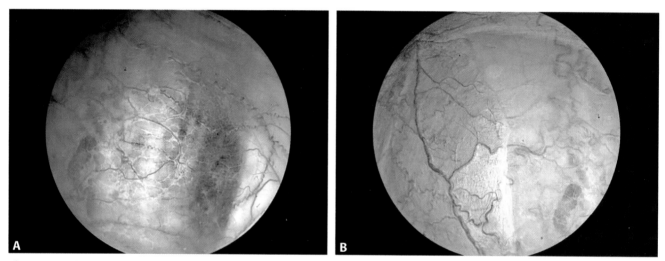

Figs. 23A and B: (A) Endoscopic view of cyst wall of patient in Figure 22. The white neural structures are seen in the right side while the darker area shows the deep midline cyst. (B) Thick cyst wall with marked vascularity. The use of YAG laser energy devascularizes the wall and minimizes bleeding.

periventricular pathology without associated ventriculomegaly, the identification of appropriate points of fenestration for the endoscopic treatment of arachnoid cysts, and in the treatment of skull base pathologies where sinus anatomy may be complex on approach and neurovascular structures are often at risk (Figs. 22 to 27).

For neuroendoscopy of the skull base, electromagnetic systems are often preferred.[14,17,19] Patient positioning during transnasal or other facial endoscopic approaches to the skull base often run into line of sight difficulties with optical-based systems. Similarly, for endoscopic-assisted approaches to the pineal region or posterior fossa pathology, electromagnetic systems are preferred. Prone positioning, even with rigid head fixation, can prove challenging for optical-based systems. In particular, while achievable, the camera can have difficulty seeing facial surface features during patient registration. Electromagnetic image guidance in such situations can allow for easier registration and intraoperative guidance. Electromagnetic systems may also be ideal in cases where rigid fixation of the head

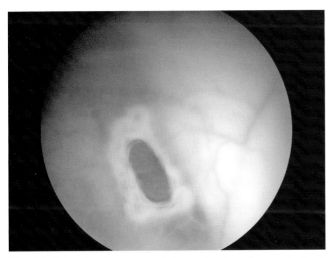

Fig. 24: Following laser coagulation of cyst wall, an ostomy is created in a bloodless fashion.

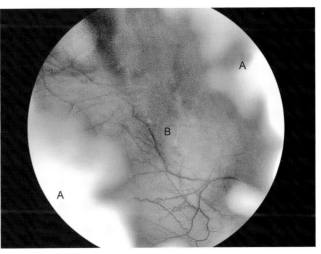

Fig. 25: Up-close view of the ostomy walls (A) shows large, deep midline cyst (B).

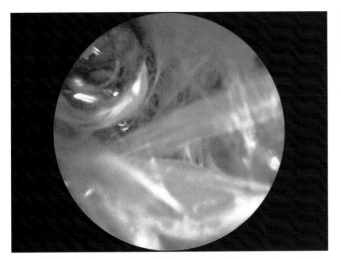

Fig. 26: Further fenestration of deep cyst wall allows fenestration and communication of the cyst with the deep arachnoid cisterns and its traversing vessels.

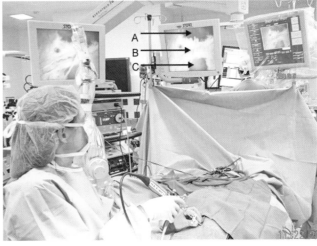

Fig. 27: Image-guided endoscopy is very useful particularly in complex cases with multiple cysts (A and C) and intervening cyst walls (B).

is desired to be avoided. Such cases may include young children or those with particular diseases of bone such as osteogenesis imperfecta.[20-22] Optical-based image guidance is preferred for endoscopic approaches to the lateral ventricles.[16] Unlike many skull base approaches, where a stylet or pointer can be placed into a position of question under direct surgeon visualization for navigation, such is not typically feasible deep within the supratentorial compartment through an endoscope introducer. In such cases the navigation of the endoscope itself is of most value.[18]

FUTURE OF INTRAOPERATIVE IMAGE-GUIDED NAVIGATION IN NEUROENDOSCOPY

Intraoperative image-guided navigation during cranial neurosurgery, including during neuroendoscopic procedures, is increasingly popular and this may be expected to expand as the technology behind intraoperative image-guided navigation continues to rapidly develop.[23] Increasingly popular is automatic registration and fusion of intraoperatively obtained images.[24] This may be pertinent with the endoscopically assisted treatment of tumors or other mass lesions where the resection itself results in brain shift and alteration compared to preoperatively obtained images. The first commercially available image guidance system based on optical pattern recognition has become available for endoscopic directed sinus surgery. Marketed by Stryker, this system requires no external patient reference array or tracking.[25,26] Instead it uses cameras attached to instruments and 3D time of flight reconstructions by a computer to determine where the instruments are located in relation to preoperatively obtained images. The technology may be portable to intraoperative image-guided navigation during neuroendoscopy. Intraoperative image-guided navigation during neuroendoscopy is an important tool for any neurosurgeon and likely to become more so as the technology continues to develop.

REFERENCES

1. Iizuka J. Development of a stereotaxic endoscopy of the ventricular system. Appl Neurophysiol. 1973;37:141-9.
2. Jacques S, Shelden H, McCann G, et al. Computerized three-dimensional stereotaxic removal of small central nervous system lesions in patients. J Neurosurg. 1980;53:816-20.
3. Leksell L, Jernberg B. Stereotaxis and tomography. A technical note. Acta Neurochir (Wien). 1980;52(1-2):1-7.
4. Hayakawa T, Tomita Y, Ikeda T, et al. A frameless, armless navigational system for computer-assisted neurosurgery. J Neurosurg. 1991;74:845-9.
5. Barnett G, Kormos D, Steiner C, et al. Use of a frameless, armless stereotactic wand for brain tumor localization with two-dimensional and three-dimensional neuroimaging. Neurosurgery. 1993;33(4):674-8.
6. Smith K, Frank K, Ducholz R. The neurostation: a highly accurate, minimally invasive solution to frameless stereotactic neurosurgery. Comput Med Imaging Graph. 1994;18(4):247-56.
7. Manwaring K, Manwaring M. Magnetic field guided endoscopic dissection through a burr hole may avoid more invasive craniotomies: a preliminary report. Minim Invasive Neurosurg II. 1994;61:34-9.
8. Goodman R. Magnetic resonance imaging-directed stereotactic endoscopic third ventriculostomy. Neurosurgery. 1993;32(6):1043-7.
9. Dorward N, Alberti O, Zhao J, et al. Interactive image-guided neuroendoscopy: development and early clinical experience. Minim Invasive Neurosurg. 1998;41(1):31-4.
10. Rhoton R, Patrick M, Luciano M, et al. Computer-assisted endoscopy for neurosurgical procedures: technical note. Neurosurgery. 1997;40(3):632-8.
11. Ryan MJ, Erickson RK, Levin DN, et al. Frameless stereotaxy with real-time tracking of patient head movement and retrospective patient-image registration. J Neurosurg. 1996;85(2):287-92.
12. Mascott CR. Comparison of magnetic tracking and optical tracking by simultaneous use of two independent frameless stereotactic systems. Neurosurgery. 2005;57(4 Suppl): 295-301.
13. Poulin F, Amiot LP. Interference during the use of an electromagnetic tracking system under OR conditions. J Biomech. 2002;35(6):733-7.
14. Hayhurst C, Byrne P, Eldridge PR, et al. Application of electromagnetic technology to neuronavigation: a revolution in image-guided neurosurgery. J Neurosurg. 2009; 111(6):1179-84.
15. Tirakotai W, Bozinov O, Sure U, et al. The evolution of stereotactic guidance in neuroendoscopy. Childs Nerv Syst. 2004;20(11-12):790-5.
16. Lee MH, Kim HR, Seol HJ, et al. Neuroendoscopic biopsy of pediatric brain tumors with small ventricle. Childs Nerv Syst. 2014;30(6):1055-60.
17. Hwang PY, Ho CL. Neuronavigation using an image-guided endoscopic transnasal-sphenoethmoidal approach to clival chordomas. Neurosurgery. 2007;61(5 Suppl 2):212-7.
18. Karabatsou K, Hayhurst C, Buxton N, et al. Endoscopic management of arachnoid cysts: an advancing technique. J Neurosurg. 2007;106(6 Suppl):455-62.
19. Mert A, Micko A, Donat M, et al. An advanced navigation protocol for endoscopic transsphenoidal surgery. World Neurosurg. 2014;82(6S):S95-S105.
20. Sangra M, Clark S, Hayhurst C, et al. Electromagnetic-guided neuroendoscopy in the pediatric population. J Neurosurg Pediatr. 2009;3(4):325-30.
21. McMillen JL, Vonau M, Wood MJ. Pinless frameless electromagnetic image-guided neuroendoscopy in children. Child's Nerv Syst. 2010;26(7):871-8.
22. Choi KY, Seo BR, Kim JH, et al. The usefulness of electromagnetic neuronavigation in the pediatric neuroendoscopic surgery. J Korean Neurosurg Soc. 2013;53(3):161-6.
23. Orringer DA, Golby A, Jolesz F. Neuronavigation in the surgical management of brain tumors: current and future trends. Expert Rev Med Devices. 2012;9(5):491-500.
24. Eggers G, Kress B, Rohde S, et al. Intraoperative computed tomography and automated registration for image-guided cranial surgery. Dentomaxillofac Radiol. 2009;38(1):28-33.
25. Mirota D, Taylor RH, Ishii M, et al. Direct endoscopic video registration for sinus surgery. In: Miga MI, Wong KH (Eds). Medical Imaging 2009: Visualization, Image-Guided Procedures, and Modeling. Bellingham: SPIE; 2009.
26. Wengert C, Székely G. Intraoperative guidance using 3D scene reconstruction from intraoperative images. In: Jolesz FA (Ed). Intraoperative Imaging and Image-Guided Therapy. New York, NY: Springer; 2014. pp. 421-38.

CHAPTER 12

Endoscopic Tumor Biopsy and Resection

David F Jimenez, David N Garza

INTRODUCTION

Intraventricular tumors remain a diagnostic and therapeutic challenge for the treating neurosurgeon. With the aid of neuroendoscopic techniques, tumor resection has become a safe, accurate, and rewarding management modality. Hydrocephalus secondary to tumor obstruction of the ventricular system aids in the management of these masses by creating a pathway for neuroendoscopic instruments. With the adjunct of neuronavigation and computer-assisted planning, a precise entry point and accurate trajectory can be planned in order to achieve maximal target accuracy. The goals of this chapter are to review the spectrum of intraventricular tumors, associated symptomatology, selection of appropriate tumors for endoscopic management, and review effectiveness and success rate of each planned procedure.

Tumors of the ventricular system arise from structures in close proximity to or within the ventricles. Most of these masses are benign but malignant types, such as metastasis, can be found in or around the ventricular system. Regardless of the tumor pathological grade, in most of the cases the immediate treatment goal consists of alleviating hydrocephalus-associated symptoms while obtaining satisfactory tissue sample in order to appropriately develop a definitive treatment plan. Tumors treated with endoscopic techniques fall into primary categories: those causing obstruction of cerebrospinal fluid (CSF) flow, i.e. blocking foramen of Monro or the aqueduct, and those present within or abutting the ventricular system without associated hydrocephalus. The goal in the former group is to restore CSF flow and obtain diagnosis, whereas the goal in latter group is both diagnosis

and resection. The specific techniques used to approach, biopsy and/or resect these lesions are described in detail in other chapters in this book.

GENERAL CONCEPTS

Ventricular neuroendoscopy can be traced back to the efforts of American urologist Victor L'Espinasse, who introduced an endoscope into the lateral ventricle of two hydrocephalic infants in 1910.[1,2] Walter Dandy attempted to incorporate the endoscope into choroid plexectomy in 1922; he also reported the first endoscopic observations of the ventricles and even coined the terms "ventriculoscope" and "ventriculoscopy".[1,3] The first modern description of endoscopic intraventricular tumor biopsy was not reported until 1973, when Takanori Fukushima et al. introduced a more flexible endoscope, the "ventriculofibroscope," for clinical use.[4] Physicians were skeptical of incorporating the endoscope into treatment planning because the technique originally had an unfavorable safety profile and low diagnostic yield.[5] However, over time, advances in optics, miniaturization, and navigation drastically improved endoscopic technology. The endoscope is now considered a simple and safe tool to implement in ventricular biopsy, tumor resection, and the hydrocephalus treatment.

Intraventricular tumors account for about 5.8% of all pediatric tumors.[6] By virtue of their location, they are often surrounded by important neural structures, such as the thalamus, the caudate nucleus, and the fornix.[7,8] A recent review conducted by Somji et al. examining 30 different neuroendoscopic biopsy studies determined that intraventricular neuroendoscopic biopsy was associated with a high diagnostic yield and relatively low rates of morbidity and mortality; the authors believe that it is reasonable to consider neuroendoscopic biopsy to be the "first-line" of therapy for the diagnosis of intraventricular lesions, particularly in cases where CSF diversion is additionally required.[5] Because intraventricular tumors often obstruct CSF pathways and bring about ventricular dilation, there is usually sufficient space for surgical positioning and maneuvering.[9] Ventriculomegaly is, generally speaking, also a favorable indicator for an endoscopic approach to tumor resection. In their 2013 intraventricular tumor resection study, Barber et al. only used neuronavigation and/or stereotactic tools when their patients lacked ventriculomegaly on preoperative imaging.[10]

Tumors originating in the ventricular system have most commonly been managed with microsurgical tools via the transcallosal or transventricular routes.[11] Complications that occur during resection, such as hemorrhage and subsequent diminished visibility, can make the neuroendoscopic approach to resection much more difficult to manage and increase the patient's risk for morbidity and mortality. In the past, because endoscopic methods lacked the ability to achieve hemostasis quickly or resect problematic tumors, microsurgery was often considered to be "the gold standard" treatment approach.[10] The gradual refinement of endoscopic tools and techniques has created better surgical outcomes and made endoscopy more accessible to physicians. However, even with the benefits of modern technology and improved technique, some surgeons still find endoscopic tumor resection to be challenging.[11]

PINEAL REGION TUMORS

Pineal region tumors are relatively rare, accounting for 0.6–0.9% of all brain tumors.[12] They are, however, significantly more common in children (10%) than adults (1–4%).[13] The symptoms most frequently seen at presentation are related to the effects of increased intracranial pressure (ICP) due to hydrocephalus: headache, nausea, vomiting, lethargy, tectal compression, and focal motor dysfunction.[14] Although there are at least 17 histologically distinct types of pineal region tumor, they can primarily be classified into four basic groups: (1) germ cell tumors, (2) pineal parenchymal tumors, (3) glial tumors, and (4) non-neoplastic masses.[15] In a paper describing their surgical experience with over 160 pineal region tumor operations,

Bruce and Stein reported that germ cell tumors were the most common type of pineal region tumor (37%), followed by glial cell tumors (28%), pineal tumors (23%), mixed tumors (15%), and spinal metastases (<10%).[16] Treatment planning for pineal region tumors is often complicated by their histological diversity, but germ cell tumors are especially susceptible to diagnostic error.[17] The incidence of these tumors also has an interesting epidemiological component that appears to be racial in nature: germ cell tumors have an incidence of 71.2% in Japan, 80% in Korea, and only 51% in Western countries.[18] Because germinoma are very radiosensitive and disproportionately distributed in the aforementioned manner, the patient populations of Japan and Korea maintained a primary treatment plan that eschewed radical surgery in favor of conservative radiotherapy for roughly a decade longer than Western populations.[18]

Although some pineal region tumors can be treated with surgical resection alone, most require either radio-therapy, chemotherapy, or both.[18] Up until the late 1970s, shunting accompanied by radiation therapy was considered the primary initial treatment for pineal region tumors because early attempts at surgery produced high rates of mortality and morbidity.[14,19] However, as microsurgical techniques improved physicians began to reevaluate surgery as a feasible approach to treatment. They were further inclined to consider surgery when some publications estimated that 36–50% of pineal tumors were benign or radioresistant and even low doses of radiation were potentially harmful to a developing brain.[14] There were also discouraging reports suggesting that ventricular shunting could contribute to the dissemination of pineal neoplasms.[20]

Because pineal region tumors are characterized by histological heterogeneity and treatment planning is so dependent on a tumor's specific histology, it is important to obtain a diagnosis via tissue biopsy before considering any specific treatment plan.[14] Neuroendoscopy is often favored as a primary approach for these cases because it enables surgeons to simultaneously obtain a safe tumor biopsy and treat symptomatic hydrocephalus without the need of a shunt or external ventricular drain. This is often a relevant advantage because reports have indicated about 90% of patients with pineal region tumors present with hydrocephalus.[15,21] In a study published by MacArthur et al., the authors determined that neuroendoscopic third ventriculostomy successfully relieved hydrocephalus in the short term for 63 out of 66 brain tumor cases (95%) and in the long-term for 55/66 tumor cases (83%).[22]

PATIENT SELECTION CRITERIA

Several authors have reported that patients diagnosed with ventriculomegaly caused by obstructive hydrocephalus are superior candidates for endoscopic surgery.[23] It has been specifically recommended that the third ventricle be one centimeter bicoronal diameter to ensure a successful surgery.[24] Enlarged ventricles are considered strong indicators for endoscopic surgery because they provide surgeons with easier access to the ventricles and more space to maneuver once they are inside. Under hydrocephalic conditions, surgeons are better able to inspect tumors for metastatic potential, circumvent injury to the choroid plexus or vascular tributaries via direct visualization, and perform multiple procedures simultaneously, if so indicated.[25] According to some authors, direct visualization also enables surgeons to obtain biopsy samples that are more likely to be "pathologically representative" of the lesion, which is thought to improve diagnostic efficacy.[26,27] Ventriculomegaly is such a strong indicator for the endoscopic approach that some surgeons insufflate patients' ventricles with 5–10 mL of lactated Ringer's solution in order to ensure that they remain open and unobstructed.[28-30]

Other authors, however, have presented evidence suggesting that the absence of hydrocephalus is not a strict contraindication for neuroendoscopic biopsy or resection. The surgeons who use neuroendoscopy under these less-than-ideal conditions often advocate the incorporation of neuronavigational tools to compensate for the diminished ventricular visibility and maneuverability of nonhydrocephalic patients.[12,28,31] In their study using neuronavigation-guided endoscopy to remove or biopsy intraventricular tumors in adult patients without hydrocephalus, Stachura and Grzywna reported that they experienced no intraoperative or postoperative complications and that none of their patients developed hydrocephalus in the long-term follow-up. Their outcomes did not greatly differ from those obtained when they treated patients who had been diagnosed with hydrocephalus.[31] Similar findings were reported in a 2014 study published by Lee et al. involving pediatric patients. The authors indicated that neuroendoscopic biopsy or resection of peri- or intraventricular tumors in pediatric patients without hydrocephalus was

feasible, but neuronavigation tools improved the accuracy of the approach and minimized brain trauma.[28]

When evaluating tumors for endoscopic resection, three important characteristics to consider are: (1) size, (2) consistency, and (3) degree of vasculature. Tumors should ideally be small (not exceeding 2–2.5 cm) soft, and avascular.[9,12] After one of their patients developed a bilateral ophthalmoplegia due to an intratumoral hematoma following the partial excision of a pineal lesion, Chibbaro et al. speculated that the endoscopic technique was not appropriate for larger, highly vascularized tumors unless gross total removal was possible.[12] Soft and/or cystic tumors are preferred because they can be debulked quickly via aspiration; rigid tumors must be dissected and removed piecemeal, which can be laborious, time-consuming, and dangerous.[10] Thankfully, the capability of surgeons to safely and successfully excise problematic tumors has been improved by the adaption and refinement of helpful surgical tools, like the ultrasonic aspirator (for larger tumors) or bipolar diathermy (for highly vascularized tumors).[9]

With regard to location, a microsurgical approach to resection has been recommended for tumors located in the fourth ventricle because of that region's limited size and precarious location; transcerebellar puncture of the fourth ventricle carries the risk of injuring the dentate nucleus.[9] With regard to patient age, a recent retrospective cohort study conducted by Bowes et al. concluded that intraventricular endoscopy was safe for pediatric patients of all ages. However, the authors also reported that the risk of endoscopic third ventriculostomy (ETV) failure and subsequent shunt placement was higher in infants, specifically those younger than 1 year of age.[32]

DIAGNOSTIC YIELD AND EFFICACY

Within the literature, the overall efficacy of neuroendoscopic intraventricular biopsy is not entirely clear. The reported rates of diagnostic yield range widely, from as low as 61% to as high as 100%.[22,33-37] This variety in yield might exist because of the differing methodological standards and practices employed by authors when reporting this information. An author's results might be further distinguished by their inclusion or exclusion of certain patient demographics, surgical characteristics, or analytical criteria. Examples might include age group, tumor type, tumor location, endoscope type, tumor forceps cup size, number of samples obtained, surgeon experience, and, most notably, the author's particular definition of "accuracy".[38] In 2008, Fiorindi and Longatti compiled several studies together and determined the overall success rate in the literature to be 88%.[39] An analysis conducted by Azab et al. in 2014 suggested that the overall percentage of biopsies that led to diagnostic information was slightly higher: 90.4%.[26] Most recently, Somji et al. conducted an analysis of 28 neuroendoscopic biopsy studies and reported the combined diagnostic yield (determined to be the percentage of samples successfully retrieved resulting in a definitive histopathologic diagnosis) to be 87.9%.[5]

While many of these numbers are promising, it should also be noted that some authors have proposed that there might be certain conditions under which endoscopic tumor biopsy (ETB) is significantly less diagnostically effective. In their paper examining the outcomes of patients undergoing endoscopic biopsy, O'Brien et al. reported that they obtained histological findings that were nondiagnostic with respect to tumor in eight of the 33 cases (24%) in which the authors performed an ETB.[23] Because seven of these cases involved pineal region tumors, the authors suggested that while ETB might be associated with fewer complications and a lower mortality rate it might also be less accurate than stereotactic biopsy in the histological diagnosis of pineal region tumors.

In 2016, Balossier et al. compared pineal tumor biopsy data from the Southampton endoscopic series40 described by Ahmed et al. in 2016 and the Lille stereotactic series[13] described by Balossier et al. in 2015. They concluded that stereotactic biopsies were ostensibly superior to endoscopic biopsies. They provided better rates of perioperative morbidity (6.4% compared to 25%), diagnosis (98.9% compared to 81.2%), accuracy (100% compared to 78.6%), and overall efficiency (98.9% compared to 63.8%).[41] Based on their findings, stereotaxis appeared, at first, be the more effective approach to pineal region tumor biopsy. However, in practice there are several instances in which the authors admit that clinical or radiological evidence would discourage the implementation of stereotactic biopsy. A diagnosis of hydrocephalus, for example, would indicate an endoscopic approach because stereotactic biopsies cannot be performed on hydrocephalic patients.[41] Robinson et al. suggested that stereotactic biopsy is further limited as an approach to

pineal region tumor biopsy because the characteristic heterogeneity of pineal region tumors increases the risk of sampling error and the surgeon's proximity to deep venous drainage systems increase the risk of hemorrhage.[20]

CLINICAL CASES

Case 1

A 67-year-old female scientist presented with chronic and progressive headaches over a several year period. She complained that she was having difficulties with memory and recalling well-established items. Additionally, she began to experience mild but bothersome ataxia. Her physical examination only showed blurred optic disks, mild dysmetria, and a positive Romberg's test. A diagnostic magnetic resonance imaging (MRI) was performed which demonstrated a brightly enhancing lesion located on the posterior third ventricle along with obstructive hydrocephalus (Figs. 1 to 4). A decision was made to obtain a biopsy via a frontal approach (Fig. 5) using image guidance (Fig. 6) and to perform an ETV via an ipsilateral coronal approach (Fig. 7). At the time of surgery, a skin incision was made on the forehead (Fig. 8) and a frontal burr hole allowed access to the frontal horn (Fig. 9). The rigid endoscope showed the foramen of Monro and the foramen was traversed to allow visualization of the

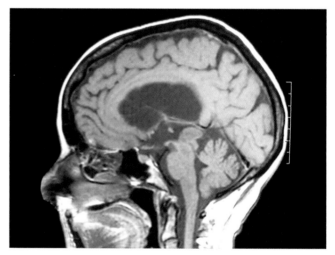

Fig. 1: Midsagittal preoperative noncontrast magnetic resonance imaging of patient in case 1 shows a heterogeneous and slightly hypointense lesion located in the pineal region area compressing the aqueduct of Sylvius and producing hydrocephalus.

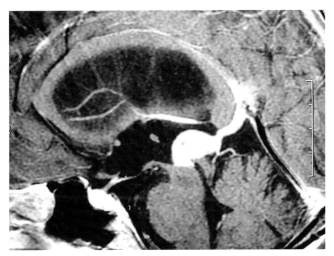

Fig. 2: Following intravenous injection of gadolinium, the lesion brightly enhanced and is well-delineated.

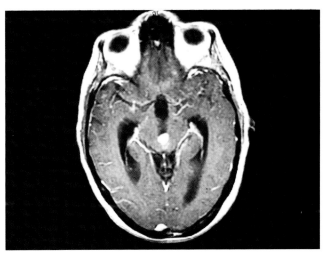

Fig. 3: Axial postcontrast magnetic resonance imaging shows the lesion abutting the posterior wall of the third ventricle.

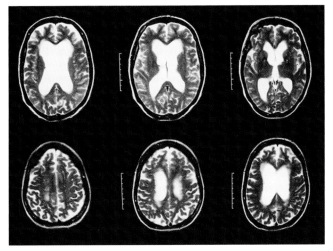

Fig. 4: T$_2$-weighted axial magnetic resonance imaging showed obstructive hydrocephalus and ventriculomegaly.

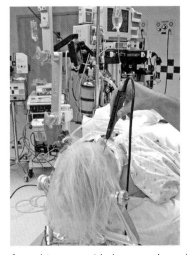

Fig. 5: A right frontal image-guided approach to the lesion was selected. Direct access to the posterior third ventricle can be easily obtained.

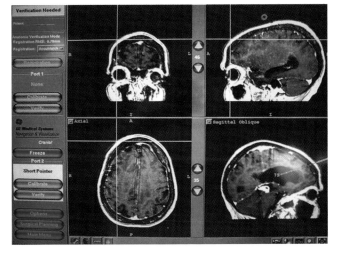

Fig. 6: A snapshot of the neuronavigation monitor shows the trajectory of the endoscope and the selected entry point.

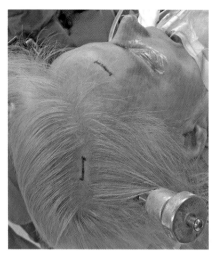

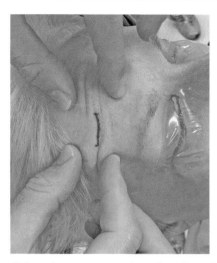

Fig. 7: The third ventriculostomy was then performed via a second coronal portal. This approach was chosen, so as to not place tension or torque on the fornix while trying to access the anterior third ventricle.

Fig. 8: A small frontal incision was selected on the right forehead to coincide with a natural forehead crease.

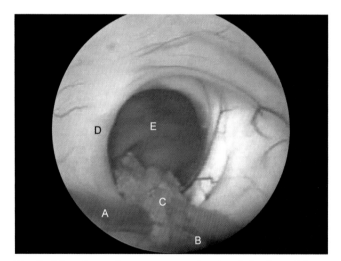

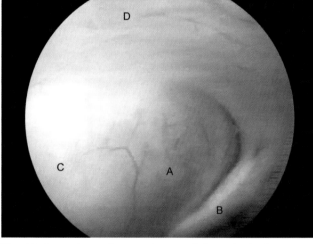

Fig. 9: After the endoscope enters the tip of the frontal horn, the following structures are easily visualized: (A) Septal vein, (B) thalamostriate vein, (C) choroid plexus, (D) fornix, and (E) foramen of Monro.

Fig. 10: Once the endoscope is passed through the foramen of Monro, the hyperpigmented lesion pushing on the wall of the third ventricle (A), the posterior commissure (B), thalamus (C), and mesencephalon (D) are seen. Note that the structures are seen upside down.

lesion (Fig. 10). The lesion was devascularized (Fig. 11) and biopsied (Fig. 12). The diagnosis was pineoblastoma. The ETV was successfully performed via a second coronal portal (Fig. 12). As early as a 4-week follow-up, the frontal incision showed superb healing (Fig. 13). The patient was treated with appropriate chemotherapy and continues to be asymptomatic and tumor-free 10 years later.

Case 2

A 22-year-old male presented with chronic headaches and fatigue. After an exhaustive workup was done, a brain MRI was done which demonstrated several brightly enhancing lesions located in the right frontal horn, left anterior hypothalamus, and posterior third ventricle. The patient

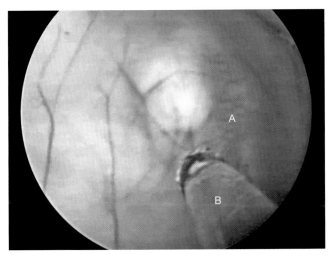

Fig. 11: The yttrium aluminum garnet (YAG) laser fiber (B) is used to devascularize the wall of the lesion (A).

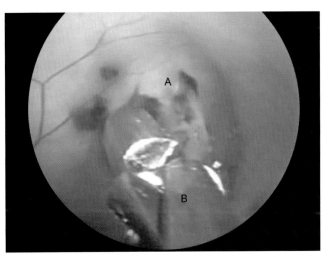

Fig. 12: The biopsy forceps (B) are used to biopsy the lesion (A).

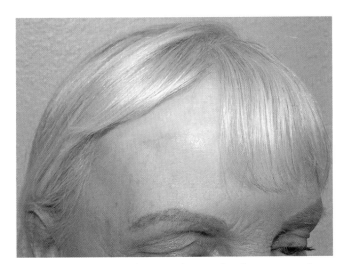

Fig. 13: Postoperative photograph 4 weeks after surgery shows superb healing of the forehead incision.

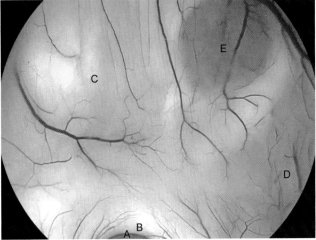

Fig. 14: Endoscopic view of right frontal horn demonstrates a metastatic germinoma (E) localized to the genu of the corpus callosum. The foramen of Monro (A) and column of the fornix (B) are visualized in the lower part of the image. The septum pellucidum (C) is seen medially and the head of the caudate nucleus (D) laterally.

also presented with mild ventriculomegaly. A decision to perform an endoscopic biopsy was done. A right frontal horn approach via a coronal burr hole was done. At the time of surgery, a brownish discolored lesion was seen on the genu of the corpus callosum (Fig. 14). Examination of the third ventricle revealed another lesion located on the anterior aspect of the left medial hypothalamus (Fig. 15). The lesion was devascularized (Fig. 16) and biopsied (Figs. 17 and 18). The diagnosis of germinoma was obtained and no further surgical resection was done. The patient was successfully discharged on postoperative day 1 and treated with chemotherapy.

Case 3

A 16-year-old right-handed female presented to the emergency room with a 3-week history of worsening generalized headaches, nausea, vomiting, ataxia and inability to eat or drink. The headaches were aggravated by activity and noise. She complained of visual difficulties with her right eye. Her neurologic and general examination were normal. A CT scan of the brain demonstrated marked

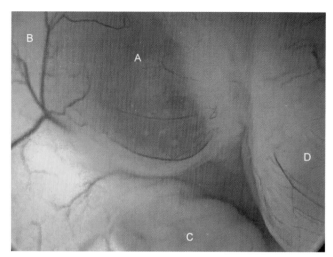

Fig. 15: The patient's close-up view of the anterior third ventricle demonstrates another germinoma lesion (A) located on the medial wall of the left hypothalamus (B). The midline tuber cinereum (C) and bulging lamina terminalis (D) are also seen.

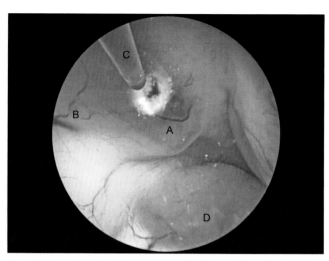

Fig. 16: A yttrium aluminum garnet (YAG) laser fiber (C) is delivering coagulating energy to the medial wall of the tumor (A). The wall is devascularized which allows for a safer biopsy. Again, the hypothalamus (B) and tuber cinereum (D) are visualized.

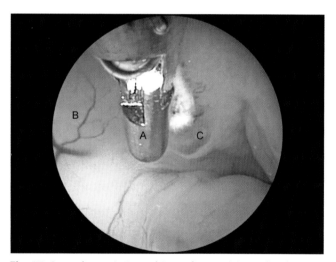

Fig. 17: An endoscopic 3 mm biopsy forceps (A) is utilized to perform the diagnostic biopsy of the germinoma (C) in the medial wall of the hypothalamus (B).

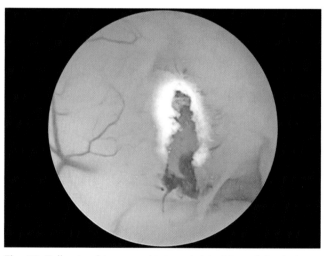

Fig. 18: Following biopsy and internal debulking of the lesion, a very small amount of blood is seen dripping from the wall of the hypothalamus. Use of the laser allows for a cleaner, less bloody biopsy.

ventriculomegaly, prominent temporal horns and a calcified lesion in the suprasellar region (Figs. 19A to D). MRI's of the brain were done which clearly demonstrated a lesion consistent with a cystic craniopharyngioma and obstructive hydrocephalus (Figs. 20A to F). She was taken to the Operating Room where an endoscopic approach to the lesion was done with image guidance via a frontal approach (Figs. 21 and 22). The third ventricular lesion was approached thru the right Foramen of Monro (Fig. 23) and the thick cyst wall was fenestrated with a laser microfiber (Fig. 24) and the cyst decompressed. The cyst wall was further coagulated and shrunk with laser and forceps (Figs. 25 and 26). The aqueduct of Sylvius was opened at the end of the case (Fig. 27). An external ventricular drain was left in for several days and removed once it was documented that she was properly

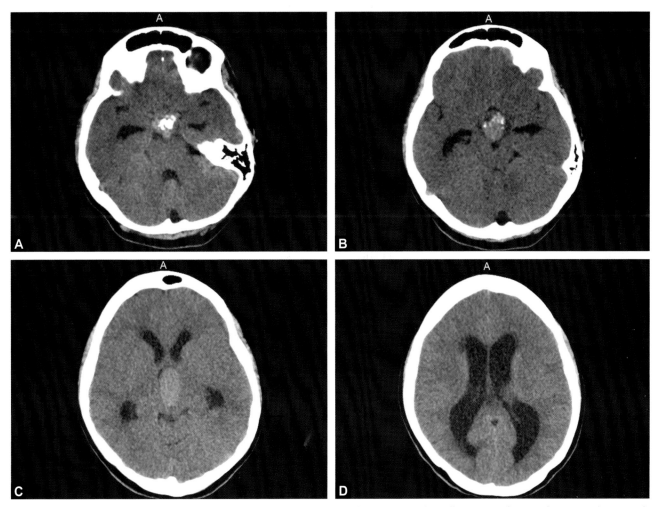

Figs. 19A to D: (A and B) Noncontrast preoperative CT scan shows calcified lesion in the sellar region along with temporal ventricular horns, indicative of hydrocephalus. (C) A hyperdense lesion is seen in the third ventricular region. (D) Marked ventricular enlargement is visualized in this preoperative CT scan.

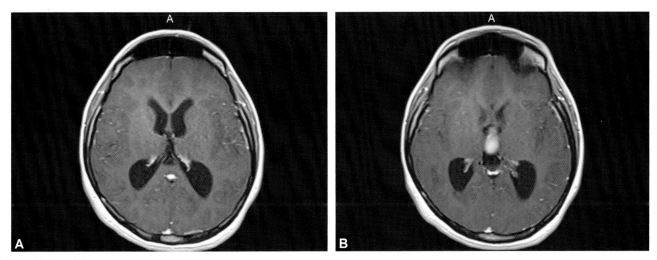

Figs. 20A and B

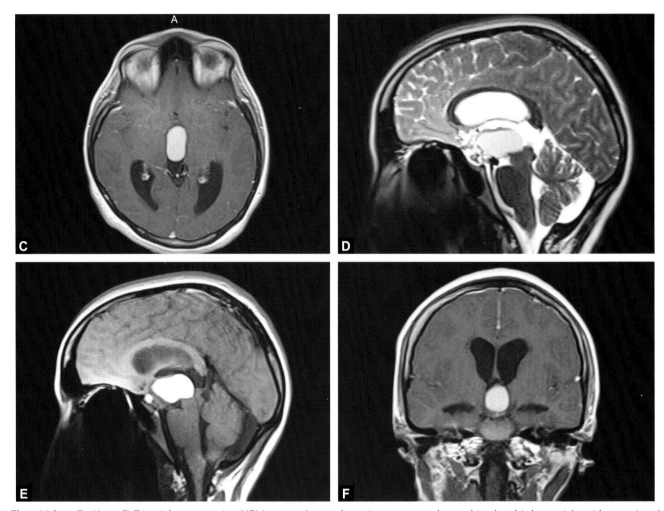

Figs. 20A to F: (A to C) T1 axial preoperative MRI images show a hyperintense mass located in the third ventricle with associated ventriculomegaly and hydrocephalus. (D and E) Sagittal MRI sequences depict a homogenous lesion filling the third ventricle which most likely represents a cyst associated with a craniopharyngioma. (F) Coronal MRI illustrating the lesion and hydrocephalus.

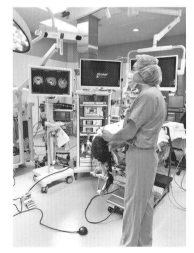

Fig. 21: Image guidance was used to properly locate the frontal entrance and to have direct access to the tip of the right frontal lobe, as seen on the images on the left side.

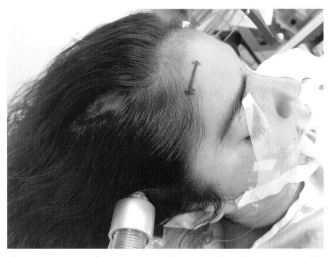

Fig. 22: A direct frontal approach was selected as seen in this photograph. An obturator cannulated the tip of the frontal horn and allowed access to the foramen of Monro.

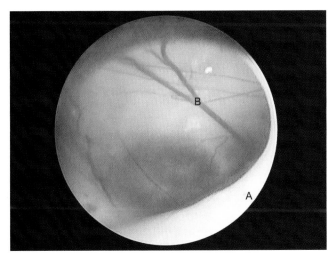

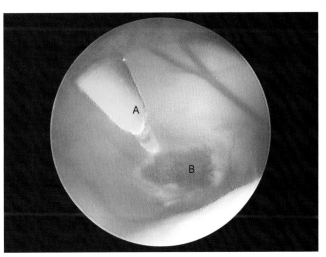

Fig. 23: Endoscopic view of the foramen of Monro shows the column of the Fornix (A) and the outer thin wall (B) of the third ventricular cyst with blood vessels running on its surface.

Fig. 24: The YAG laser fiber (A) is being used to create a fenestration (B) on the cyst wall.

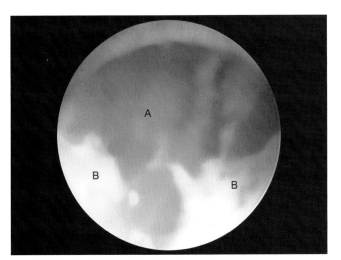

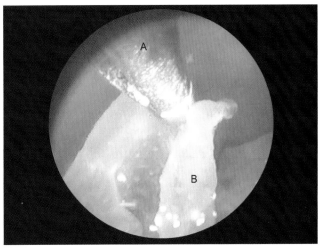

Fig. 25: The green liquid material inside the cyst is seen extruding through the fenestrated (B) cyst.

Fig. 26: A graping forceps (A) is being used to remove the thicker inner wall (B) of the cyst.

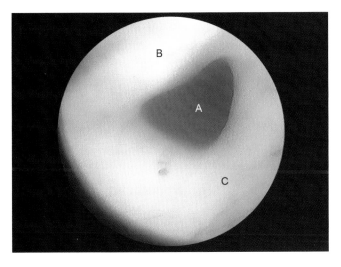

Fig. 27: After removal of the cyst contents from the third ventricle, an open aqueduct of Sylvius (A) is visualized as well as the posterior commisure (B) and the mesencephalon (C) which makes the floor of the posterior third ventricle.

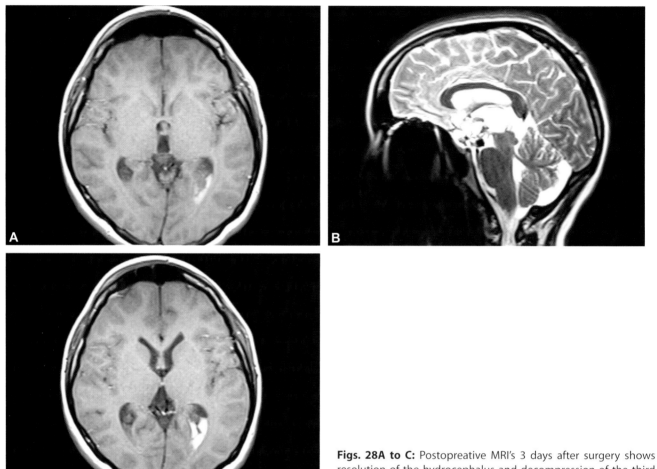

Figs. 28A to C: Postopreative MRI's 3 days after surgery shows resolution of the hydrocephalus and decompression of the third ventricle with cyst removal. The patient was asymptomatic.

absorbing her CSF and had normal ICP's. Postoperative scans showed adequate ventricular decompression and the patient became asymptomatic (Figs. 28A to C).

Technical Considerations

Appropriate burr hole placement is the most important step in any endoscopic procedure (*see* Figs. 4, 6 to 9, 11, 13 to 16 of Chapter 4). When planning an ETV, a standard precoronal burr hole should be considered, taking into consideration anatomical variability, such as massa inter-media, when planning trajectory. However, each case should be carefully planned using triplanar MRI images in order to plan the best and most direct access to the anterior third ventricle. Often times the burr hole needs to be placed slightly anterior to the coronal suture along the mid-pupillary line especially for pineal region tumors

and posterior third ventricular tumors. When using rigid endoscopes, a skin incision can be made on the forehead, on one of the skin creases. This allows direct access to the posterior third ventricle and can be achieved through the foramen of Monro.[2,6,8,20] When planning a septostomy, the burr hole should be more lateral allowing a direct view of the septum.[8] Those are important factors to consider in order to achieve a high diagnostic yield for tumor biopsies. This also applies to success of ETV with appropriate burr hole placement planning.

Endoscopy should always be considered in patients requiring a CSF diversion procedure due to tumor obstructive hydrocephalus (ETV and/or septostomy). Endoscopy remains the absolute tool to obtain safe minimally invasive tumor specimen to help institute appropriate treatment/adjuvant treatment. Understanding the patient's anatomy and anatomical limitations (massa intermedia, unfavorable floor of the third ventricle, and basilar artery tortuosity) is crucial in keeping this procedure safe and achieving the best outcome possible

COMPLICATIONS AND RECOMMENDATIONS

In the literature, the reported complication rates for intraventricular tumor resection vary greatly, from 0–20.8%.[10,30,42,43] The most frequently mentioned complications for endoscopic management are: intraoperative bleeding, postoperative residual tumor apoplexy, ventricular collapse, pneumocephalus, and tumor dissemination.[44] Gaab and Schroeder reported that small hemorrhages occur during nearly all tumor resections and biopsies; they are problematic because even a small amount of bleeding can obscure operative visualization.[8] Surgeons are advised to maintain continuous irrigation with sufficient outflow, ensure that they have a large working channel, and cauterize large vessels that are at risk for hemorrhage before tumor dissection is attempted.[9] If bleeding persists or becomes significant, it can be stemmed by implementing bipolar diathermy.[8] For gross total resection, the most frequently cited complications accompanying neuroendoscopy are: hemorrhage (intraventricular and/or intraparenchymal), infections (ventriculitis and/or meningitis) neuropsychological deficit, CSF leak, infarction, cranial nerve deficit, and hormonal disturbance.[42]

Because there is evidence of a higher risk for colloid cyst recurrence after endoscopic resection when compared to microsurgical resection, some authors have speculated that tumors resected endoscopically are more likely recur than those resected via microsurgery.[45] However, more studies conducted over the long-term are needed before such conclusions can be definitive. The reported recurrence rates for microsurgical resection vary greatly within the literature and recurrence itself seems to be dependent on a wide range of factors, including: tumor type, resection completion, and the use of adjuvant therapies.[10] It has generally advised that if a surgeon is planning to perform both an ETB and an ETV, the ETV should be performed last. If third ventriculostomy is performed first, there is a possibility that the tumor will bleed and spread throughout the subarachnoid space, which can ultimately lead to the development of communicating hydrocephalus.[46] If the biopsy is performed first, it might help the surgeon avoid tumor seeding via irrigation of the ventricular space.[46]

When Azab et al. conducted a review of endoscopic brain biopsy within the medical literature, they concluded that surgeries performed with rigid lenscopes had a higher diagnostic yield than those performed by flexible fiberscopes (93.54% vs 74.76).[26] A rigid instrument are thought to offer superior optical and light quality in addition to superior instrument control and manipulation; these advantages might enable surgeons to obtain larger quantities of pathological tissue during biopsies, preserve neural structures during surgery, remove tumors more efficiently, and maintain hemostasis.[12] Although rigid endoscopes allow for better tumor visualization, their reduced maneuverability could also make it more difficult for surgeons to access posterior tumors.[41] However, the value placed on these advantages and disadvantages is still being contested within the literature. In their comprehensive review of neuroendoscopic biopsies, Somji et al. determined that there was not a significant difference in diagnostic yield when they compared studies that exclusively used rigid or flexible endoscopes.[5]

When surgeons discuss the endoscopic approach for patients with less than ideal anatomical structure, they sometimes recommend neuronavigation tools as a way to compensate for diminished visibility or maneuverability. As a result of these recommendations, there has been some debate within the literature about whether neuronavigation should routinely accompany neuroendoscopy, or if it would be more practical to limit it to select cases. In their prospective clinical series, Rohde et al. determined that neuronavigation was valuable in more than 50% of the cases they reviewed.[47] However, that value varied according procedure. Neuronavigation seemed to be most useful when it assisted surgeons performing tumor biopsies, tumor resections, and cyst fenestration; it was least helpful when used in conjunction with an ETV.[47] The authors ultimately concluded that the routine inclusion of neuronavigation was advisable because it minimized the need for anatomical landmarks and enabled surgeons to define the best trajectory, overcome poor visualization, and identify obscured or hidden structures. Preoperative MRI can sometimes be used beforehand to identify patients for whom neuronavigation might be helpful, but it is unable to detect thickening and opacity of the third ventricular floor.[47]

CONCLUSION

Endoscopic techniques are a very useful adjunct to the neurosurgeon treating ventricular lesions associated with hydrocephalus. As a first step, diagnosis can be obtained and CSF can be restored. Once diagnosis is obtained further determination as to the best therapeutic modality can be established: microsurgical resection, chemotherapy, or radiotherapy, if indicated. Careful planning and execution are essential for a successful clinical outcome.

REFERENCES

1. Decq P, Schroeder HW, Fritsch M, et al. A history of ventricular neuroendoscopy. World Neurosurg. 2013;79:S14. e1-6.

2. Doglietto F, Prevedello DM, Jane JA Jr, et al. Brief history of endoscopic transsphenoidal surgery—from Philipp Bozzini to the First World Congress of Endoscopic Skull Base Surgery. Neurosurg Focus. 2005;19:E3.

3. Hellwig D, Grotenhuis JA, Tirakotai W, et al. Endoscopic third ventriculostomy for obstructive hydrocephalus. Neurosurg Rev. 2005;28:1-34.

4. Fukushima T, Ishijima B, Hirakawa K, et al. Ventriculofiberscope: a new technique for endoscopic diagnosis and operation. J Neurosurg. 1973;38:251-6.

5. Somji M, Badhiwala J, McLellan A, et al. Diagnostic yield, morbidity, and mortality of intraventricular neuroendoscopic biopsy: systematic review and meta-analysis. World Neurosurg. 2016;85:315-24.e2.

6. Ostrom QT, Gittleman H, Farah P, et al. CBTRUS statistical report: Primary brain and central nervous system tumors diagnosed in the United States in 2006-2010. Neuro Oncol. 2013;15:ii1-ii56.

7. Morita A, Kelly PJ. Resection of intraventricular tumors via a computer-assisted volumetric stereotactic approach. Neurosurgery. 1993;32:920-6; discussion 926-7.

8. Gaab MR, Schroeder HW. Neuroendoscopic approach to intraventricular lesions. Neurosurgical focus. 1999;6(4):e5.

9. Schroeder HW. Intraventricular tumors. World Neurosurg. 2013;79:S17.e15-9.

10. Barber SM, Rangel-Castilla L, Baskin D. Neuroendoscopic resection of intraventricular tumors: a systematic outcomes analysis. Minim Invasive Surg. 2013;2013:898753.

11. Kim MH. Transcortical Endoscopic Surgery for Intraventricular Lesions. J Korean Neurosurg Soc. 2017;60: 327-34.

12. Chibbaro S, Di Rocco F, Makiese O, et al. Neuroendoscopic management of posterior third ventricle and pineal region tumors: technique, limitation, and possible complication avoidance. Neurosurg Rev. 2012;35:331-8; discussion 338-40.

13. Balossier A, Blond S, Touzet G, et al. Endoscopic versus stereotactic procedure for pineal tumour biopsies: comparative review of the literature and learning from a 25-year experience. Neurochirurgie. 2015;61:146-54.

14. Edwards MS, Hudgins RJ, Wilson CB, et al. Pineal region tumors in children. J Neurosurg. 1988;68:689-97.

15. Schild SE, Scheithauer BW, Schomberg PJ, et al. Pineal parenchymal tumors: clinical, pathologic, and therapeutic aspects. Cancer. 1993;72:870-80.

16. Bruce JN, Stein BM. Surgical management of pineal region tumors. Acta Neurochir (Wien). 1995;134:130-5.

17. Kinoshita Y, Yamasaki F, Tominaga A, et al. Pitfalls of Neuroendoscopic Biopsy of Intraventricular Germ Cell Tumors. World Neurosurg. 2017;106:430-4.

18. Oi S, Shibata M, Tominaga J, et al. Efficacy of neuroendoscopic procedures in minimally invasive preferential management of pineal region tumors: a prospective study. J Neurosurg. 2000;93:245-53.

19. Oi S, Matsuzawa K, Choi JU, et al. Identical characteristics of the patient populations with pineal region tumors in Japan and in Korea and therapeutic modalities. Childs Nerv Syst. 1998;14:36-40.

20. Robinson S, Cohen AR. The role of neuroendoscopy in the treatment of pineal region tumors. Surg Neurol. 1997; 48:360-5.

21. Gangemi M, Maiuri F, Colella G, et al. Endoscopic surgery for pineal region tumors. min-Minim Invasive Neurosurg. 2001;44:70-3.

22. Macarthur DC, Buxton N, Punt J, et al. The role of neuroendoscopy in the management of brain tumours. Br J Neurosurg. 2002;16:465-70.

23. O'Brien DF, Hayhurst C, Pizer B, et al. Outcomes in patients undergoing single-trajectory endoscopic third ventriculostomy and endoscopic biopsy for midline tumors presenting with obstructive hydrocephalus. J Neurosurg. 2006; 105:219-26.

24. Jones RF, Stening WA, Brydon M. Endoscopic third ventriculostomy. Neurosurgery. 1990;26:86-91; discussion 91-2.

25. Souweidane MM. Endoscopic surgery for intraventricular brain tumors in patients without hydrocephalus. Neurosurgery. 2005;57:312-8; discussion 312-8.

26. Azab WA, Nasim K, Chelghoum A, et al. Endoscopic biopsy of brain tumors: Does the technique matter? Surg Neurol Int. 2014;5:159.

27. Chowdhry SA, Cohen AR. Intraventricular neuroendoscopy: complication avoidance and management. World Neurosurg. 2013;79:S15.e1-10.

28. Lee MH, Kim HR, Seol HJ, et al. Neuroendoscopic biopsy of pediatric brain tumors with small ventricle. Childs Nerv Syst. 2014;30:1055-60.

29. Cappabianca P, Cinalli G, Gangemi M, et al. Application of neuroendoscopy to intraventricular lesions. Neurosurgery. 2008;62:575-97; discussion 597-8.

30. Naftel RP, Shannon CN, Reed GT, et al. Small-ventricle neuroendoscopy for pediatric brain tumor management. J Neurosurg Pediatr. 2011;7:104-10.

31. Stachura K, Grzywna E. Neuronavigation-guided endoscopy for intraventricular tumors in adult patients without hydrocephalus. Wideochir Inne Tech Maloinwazyjne. 2016;11:200-7.

32. Bowes AL, King-Robson J, Dawes WJ, et al. Neuroendoscopic surgery in children: does age at intervention influence

safety and efficacy? A single-center experience. J Neurosurg Pediatr. 2017;20:324-8.

33. Ahn ES, Goumnerova L. Endoscopic biopsy of brain tumors in children: diagnostic success and utility in guiding treatment strategies. J Neurosurg Pediatr. 2010;5:255-62.

34. Depreitere B, Dasi N, Rutka J, et al. Endoscopic biopsy for intraventricular tumors in children. J Neurosurg. 2007; 106:340-6.

35. Tirakotai W, Hellwig D, Bertalanffy H, et al. The role of neuroendoscopy in the management of solid or solid-cystic intra- and periventricular tumours. Childs Nerv Syst. 2007;23:653-8.

36. Shono T, Natori Y, Morioka T, et al. Results of a long-term follow-up after neuroendoscopic biopsy procedure and third ventriculostomy in patients with intracranial germinomas. J Neurosurg. 2007;107:193-8.

37. Prat R, Galeano I. Endoscopic biopsy of foramen of Monro and third ventricle lesions guided by frameless neuronavigation: usefulness and limitations. Clin Neurol Neurosurg. 2009;111:579-82.

38. Giannetti AV, Alvarenga AY, de Lima TO, et al. Neuroendoscopic biopsy of brain lesions: accuracy and complications. J Neurosurg. 2015;122:34-9.

39. Fiorindi A, Longatti P. A restricted neuroendoscopic approach for pathological diagnosis of intraventricular and paraventricular tumours. Acta Neurochir (Wien). 2008;150:1235-9.

40. Ahmed AI, Zaben MJ, Mathad NV, et al. Endoscopic biopsy and third ventriculostomy for the management of pineal region tumors. World Neurosurg. 2015;83:543-7.

41. Balossier A, Blond S, Reyns N. Endoscopic versus stereo-tactic procedure for pineal tumor biopsies: focus on overall efficacy rate. World Neurosurg. 2016;92:223-8.

42. Hidalgo ET, Ali A, Weiner HL, et al. Resection of intraventricular tumors in children by purely endoscopic means. World Neurosurg. 2016;87:372-80.

43. Cinalli G, Spennato P, Ruggiero C, et al. Complications following endoscopic intracranial procedures in children. Childs Nerv Syst. 2007;23:633-44.

44. Chibbaro S, Champeaux C, Poczos P, et al. Anterior transfrontal endoscopic management of colloid cyst: an effective, safe, and elegant way of treatment. Case series and technical note from a multicenter prospective study. Neurosurg Rev. 2014;37:235-41; discussion 241.

45. Horn EM, Feiz-Erfan I, Bristol RE, et al. Treatment options for third ventricular colloid cysts: comparison of open microsurgical versus endoscopic resection. Neurosurgery. 2007;62:1076-83.

46. Yurtseven T, Erşahin Y, Demirtaş E, et al. Neuroendoscopic biopsy for intraventricular tumors. Minim Invasive Neurosurg. 2003;46:293-9.

47. Rohde V, Behm T, Ludwig H, et al. The role of neuronavigation in intracranial endoscopic procedures. Neurosurg Rev. 2012;35:351-8.

CHAPTER 13

Endoscopic Microvascular Decompression

David F Jimenez, David N Garza

INTRODUCTION

Trigeminal neuralgia (TN) is the most common facial neuralgia, with an overall crude incidence rate of 4.3 per 100,000 per year.[1,2] The study of TN can be traced back to the late 1920s and early 1930s when Dandy identified the frequent compression of lesions (such as tumors, arteries, or veins) against the trigeminal nerve root.[3] Later, in 1962, Gardner concluded that these compressions can cause demyelination and create a "short circuit" between the touch and pain fibers; the action current of the evoked afferent barrage, transmitted by sensory root fibers upon reaching the point of compression, excites pain fibers of similar size and conduction rate.[4] In 1967, Kerr visualized trigeminal root demyelination in patients with TN using light and electron microscopes. He affirmed the idea that segmental demyelination might be responsible for producing the short-circuiting spots Gardner described where ephaptic transmissions provoked paroxysmal pain.[3,5] Around that same time, Jannetta proposed that blood vessels (most frequently aberrant arteries) were the structures compressing the dorsal root entry zone (Fig. 1). By decompressing the trigeminal root, permanent relief of paroxysmal pain could be achieved without destroying any neural tissue.[3] Jannetta standardized this operation when he published his 1967 paper describing a microvascular decompression (MVD) via the subtemporal transtentorial route (Fig. 2).[6] MVD subsequently became the treatment of choice for TN because of its high incidence

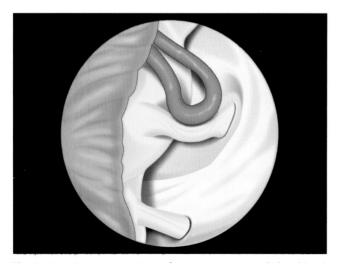

Fig. 1: Artistic representation of Jannetta's proposal that blood vessels decompressed the root entry zone of cranial nerve V to produce trigeminal neuralgia.

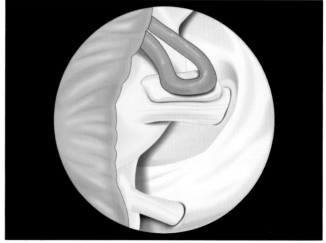

Fig. 2: Artist's rendition of Jannetta's surgical procedure of decompressing the trigeminal nerve and relief of neuralgia.

of long-term relief, its low recurrence of pain rate, and the fact that it was unlikely to engender sensory changes.[3]

Microvascular decompression has been modified in recent years to include endoscopic exploration and decompression. The endoscopic approach has permitted the management of neural-vascular conflicts without extensive surgical dissection or retraction and aided in the visualization of the cerebellopontine angle vasculature with greater detail than microscopy alone.[1,7] Endoscopy increases the clarity of the surgical field and simultaneously achieves panoramic visualization, which helps the surgeon locate sites of neurovascular conflict and accurately assess decompression without increasing invasiveness.[1,8-10] Sandell et al. recently reported that the endoscope significantly aided the identification of neurovascular conflict in their TN patients, particularly in cases where a bony ridge posterior to the trigeminal nerve (suprameatal tubercle) obscured the view of the vessel(s) compressing the fifth nerve.[11] Rak et al. reported similar results in their study. They wrote that the endoscope was especially useful in identifying trigeminal vein compression of cranial nerve V in Meckel's cave, cranial nerve VII at the root exit zone, and cranial nerve VIII in patients with TN, hemifacial spasm, and disabling positional vertigo.[12] The endoscope can be an invaluable tool, but it requires an experienced hand to wield it effectively. Due to a lack of depth perception, simulator-operative training is recommended for those individuals who might be new to endoscopic approaches.[1]

In addition to endoscope-assisted MVD, there is also endoscopic vascular decompression (EVD), in which microscopy is not used at all; the entire process is performed using only endoscopic tools. Jarrahy et al. pioneered EVD in 2002 when they published their study describing the use of an endoscope as the exclusive imaging modality for trigeminal nerve decompression. They concluded that the endoscope provided superior visualization that aided in identifying neurovascular conflicts and evaluating the thoroughness of decompression.[13] EVD is reported to have several other benefits, including a smaller craniotomy, less soft tissue dissection, less cerebellar retraction, no extensive dissection (which is often required for microscopic exposure), and faster patient recovery.[7,13] It is safe, highly effective, and offers results that are comparable to both traditional MVD and endoscope-assisted MVD.[7]

Although MVD and its derivative treatments are helpful in alleviating many patients' symptoms, TN patients do not always have observable vascular compression.[14] The estimated incidence of this phenomenon varies from 3.5% to 8.7%, although it is possible that supposedly negative results from surgical exploration can be attributed to a lack of experience on the surgeon's part, especially when the vascular conflict is located in the cerebellopontine angle.[3,15] In the absence of vascular compression, other anatomical factors that could influence the development of TN include global root atrophy, focal arachnoid thickening, and a ribbon-shaped angulated root crossing over the petrous ridge.[6] Some authors maintain that cerebral atrophy and arteriosclerosis are fundamental conditions for the development of TN, but that supposition would not account for the young patients who have TN that do not share these characteristics.[15] Performing trigeminal root compression can still provide some initial relief to these patients, but the long-term efficacy, complication rates, and recurrence rates are unsatisfactory.[16] Because it is apparent neurovascular conflict is not the sole causative factor, many authors believe that more studies should be conducted and different treatment possibilities for TN should be explored.

One possible surgical alternative to MVD is a partial sensory rhizotomy (PSR), which involves lesioning the sensory trigeminal nerve root. In a study conducted by Young and Wilkins, PSR demonstrated a 70% success rate in which patients had excellent or good outcomes after an average follow-up period of 72 months.[17] However, an inevitable side effect of that procedure is sensory loss and potential side effects include deafferentation pain, keratitis, and eating difficulties.[18] Other surgical alternatives exist as well, including as balloon rhizotomy, glycerol injections, and radiosurgery.[14] Because there is not yet a consensus regarding which treatment is the best to implement in cases without vascular conflict, it is recommended that surgeons optimize preoperative imaging in order to determine the ideal surgical candidates for the various types of intervention currently available.[16]

LITERATURE REVIEW

The success of MVD is dependent on the surgeon's ability to survey the operational field, identify any compressing vessels, and execute effective decompression. Endoscopic assistance is capable of improving performance in all these areas by enhancing visualization. In 2000, Jarrahy et al. recorded some of the first descriptions of endoscopy being implemented as an adjunctive imaging modality to microscopy. Within their study of 21 patients with TN, they identified 51 nerve-vessel conflicts. Of those 51 conflicts, 14 (27%) were in areas inaccessible to microscopic visualization; they could only be detected endoscopically.[10] Similar findings were reported by Teo et al. in 2006 and Chen et al. in 2008. In Teo's study examining 113 TN patients who underwent endoscope-assisted MVD, endoscopy revealed arteries in 38 patients (33%) that were poorly seen or not seen at all with a microscope.[19] In Chen's study of 167 patients, 23 (14.74%) had conflicts that had been missed by the microscope.[1]

Endoscopic approaches to MVD might also enhance the long-term efficacy of surgical intervention for TN. A study conducted by Barker et al. regarding 1,185 patients who had undergone traditional, open MVD determined that complete, immediate postoperative relief was experienced in 82% of patients; 1 year later, among 1,155 patients that were followed, the percentage who still had complete pain relief dropped to 75%.[20] By comparison, after a mean follow-up period of 29 months in Teo's study, 112 of their 113 patients who had successfully undergone endoscope-assisted MVD (99.1%) still experienced complete pain relief.[19] In 2005, Kabil et al. studied 255 patients who had undergone endoscopic vascular decompression. The authors noted an initial, complete, postoperative success rate of 95% for the 255 patient population and documented a 93% complete success rate in 118 patients who participated in at least a 3-year follow-up.[21]

Since 1980, there has been much speculation about how to accurately predict the long-term outcome of MVD for TN. Many variables have been considered in an effort to determine what factors might be associated with TN recurrence, including the onset of pain, type of pain, presentation of pain (typical or atypical), presence of facial trigger points, type of vascular compression, degree of vascular conflict, duration of symptoms, immediate postoperative outcome, previous MVD surgical history, and even patient sex.[20,22-27] The factors most frequently discussed in the literature involve the presentation of the patient's pain or the characteristics of their vascular conflict at the time of surgery.

In 1988, Burchiel et al. observed a strong statistical relationship between arterial cross-compression of the nerve and long-term, complete pain relief. They proposed that the source of the vascular compression was a significant factor in determining MVD outcomes.[22] In their study, four out of seven patients with venous compression

(57%) experienced major pain recurrence, while only six out of 25 patients with arterial nerve impingement (24%) experienced a similar recurrence.[22] In the early 1990s, Sun et al. affirmed Burchiel's findings when they reported that venous compression (singly or in combination with arteries) was significantly associated with recurrence. In their study, recurrence was seen in four out of five (80%) venous compression cases, and only six out of 51 (11%) arterial compression cases.[26] Similar observations were made by Barker et al. in 1996 and Li et al. in 2004. Barker's study determined that venous compression of the trigeminal root was a significant predictive factor for TN recurrence.[20] Li et al. reported that single artery compression was often associated with better patient outcomes. Out of 62 patients Li et al. studied only 11 with some degree of vein compression achieved pain relief. By comparison, the authors observed 49 patients with only artery compression who achieved significant pain relief.[23]

Dahle et al. also believed long-term pain remission was related to the characteristics of the vascular compression encountered during surgery. However, they asserted that it was not the type of vessel or vessels involved in the conflict that was important as much as the degree of compression created by those vessels. They followed up 54 MVD patients 3.1 years after surgery and found that the cases with combined arterial and venous compression experienced a pain relief rate of 100% (16 out of 16 cases) compared to rates of 75% (21 out of 28 cases) for pure arterial and 60% (6 out of 10 cases) for pure venous compression.[27] They contended that it was not vessel type, venous or arterial, but an increase in compression created by a combination of vessels that truly predicted a pain-free outcome.

In 2007, Sindou et al. conducted a study in which 362 patients who had undergone MVD for TN were followed up over a period of one to 18 years. The authors reported that although pure venous compression cases had a lower success rate at the 15 year mark compared to arterial compression cases, the finding was not statistically significant.[25] Instead, like Dahle et al., they suggested that it was the severity of vascular compression that mattered most when determining the risk of recurrence. In their study, the authors saw 350 cases of arterial compression; they assessed the severity of their neurovascular conflict and assigned a rating to them on a scale of I to III. At the 1 year and 15-year follow-up, patients assigned with a degree III compression had cure rates of 96.6% and 88.1% respectively, those with degree II compressions had rates of 90.2% and 78.3%, and those with degree I compressions had rates of 83.3% and 58.3%.[25] With arterial compression cases, both in the short-term and long-term, the more aggressive the degree of preoperative compression, the better was the patient's chances for a pain-free outcome.

With regard to the characterization of pain, many authors have observed a difference between typical and atypical TN patient outcomes. For the most part, it appears as if typical patients have better chances at achieving both short-term and long-term relief. In a study conducted by Tyler-Kabara et al., 2,675 TN cases (2003 typical and 672 atypical) were reviewed to assess immediate, postoperative pain relief, 1,188 of which (969 typical and 219 atypical) had follow-up data for more than 5 years that was also evaluated to assess long-term pain relief.[28] For the typical TN patients, 80.3% achieved excellent, immediate postoperative relief, 16.5% achieved good (partial) relief, and 3.2% had no response; for the long-term follow-up, 73.7% achieved excellent pain relief, 6.8% had good pain relief, and 19.5% had no long-term pain relief.[28] Among atypical patients, 46.9% achieved excellent, immediate postoperative relief, 39.7% achieved good relief, and 13.4% had no response; for the long-term follow-up, 34.7% had excellent pain relief, 16.4% had good pain relief, and 48.9% experienced no pain relief.[28]

Like Tyler-Kabara et al., several other authors have noted this apparent relationship between pain presentation and patient outcomes. In their study, Li et al. reported that among 13 atypical patients the rate of complete pain relief was 29.4%, but in 45 patients with typical TN presentation, the rate of postoperative complete pain relief was 97.8%.[23] Miller et al. believed that typical TN was associated with favorable outcomes because, in their study, pain relief after MVD was strongly correlated with the lancinating pain component.[24] In fact, Miller et al. concluded that the type of pain presented by the patient more accurately predicted surgical outcome than any other feature of TN. This lends some credence to the theory that the different types of TN are not actually discrete diagnoses; they might instead represent different points along the same continuous spectrum of injury. If that model is accurate, it is possible that atypical TN cases experience worse surgical outcomes than typical cases because constant (rather than lancinating) pain actually indicates that the patient is suffering from a more advanced trigeminal neuropathy rather than an entirely separate etiology.[24] It should be noted, however, that not

all authors have encountered the same findings regarding typical TN presentation or lancinating pain. According to Sindou's MVD study, the characteristics of patient presentation did not appear to play any role in prognosis. Atypical TN cases had approximately the same cure rates as those with typical neuralgia at both one year and 15-year follow-up periods.[25]

There are several other potentially predictive factors related to a patient's presentation of TN. Barker et al. maintained that symptoms lasting less than 8 years and immediate postoperative relief both predicted long-term pain relief after MVD.[20] Li's study concluded that a shorter symptom duration (especially not longer than 3 years) and an unchanging distribution of facial pain predicted a better operative outcome.[23] Tyler-Kabara et al. reported that the presence of trigger points and a memorable onset of pain predicted immediate, postoperative pain relief for both typical and atypical cases; the presence of trigger points predicted a better long-term outcome as well, but only for typical TN cases.[28] The location of the patient's pain can also change and become bilateral at some stage in the disease; this happens for between 5% and 10% of patients, sometimes after surgical intervention.[15] Because the pathology of TN is complex and still debated, it is possible that all these factors could be relevant, in some way, to the prediction of postoperative outcomes. Based on these findings, we can develop a general guideline for surgical selection. The ideal candidate for MVD surgery might be a person who has a short history of lancinating pain with specific trigger points and severe, arterial vascular compression. His or her long-term success is especially probable if there was a memorable onset of pain and immediate relief after surgical intervention. Should that patient end up experiencing recurrent pain, Gu et al. recently reported that an initial, prolonged, pain-free period following surgery can be considered an encouraging indication for revisiting MVD in cases of recurrent TN.[29]

CLINICAL PRESENTATION

Trigeminal neuralgia typically presents as a unilateral, lancinating, paroxysmal pain in one or more of the trigeminal nerve distributions.[1,28] The pain might occur spontaneously, be triggered by touching or moving the face, air hitting the face, brushing the teeth, or be positional in nature. Atypical TN pain is also unilateral, but it is more often described as a burning or aching rather than piercing. It may be continuous (or nearly continuous) and will rarely respond to medication.[28] The typical form might evolve into the atypical form over many years and, during that process, a patient might experience a third "transitional TN" stage that has characteristics of both typical and atypical TN.[28] Each episode of typical or "classic" TN generally lasts between a few seconds to several minutes; intermittent periods of remission, when a patient is pain-free and displays no symptoms, can span months or even years before a relapse occurs.[20,28] Pain-free intervals usually grow shorter in duration and eventually disappear.[20] Typical TN patients often experience some relief with medication, such as carbamazepine, phenytoin, or baclofen, but the potency of those drugs can decrease over time or produce undesirable side effects.[20,28] Under those circumstances, a patient would likely be considered a candidate for surgical intervention.

SURGICAL PROCEDURE

Preoperative Considerations

An appropriate preoperative medical workup and clearance for surgery is obtained. Neuronavigation is a valuable tool in assuring that the burr hole is appropriately placed and as such a preoperative MRI is obtained with neuronavigational protocol. As it is with the majority of the cases, the MRI will not likely demonstrate a specific vascular compression of the trigeminal nerve. Occasionally, a large ectatic vertebral artery may be seen at or near the root entry zone (Figs. 3A and B). Care should

be taken to make sure that all endoscopic instruments are available and the endoscopic system is properly working. This procedure calls for a two-handed approach as would a microscopic approach. Therefore, the challenge lies on how to manipulate the visualizing endoscope. It is best to free hand the endoscope during the early visualization of the surgical field and the cerebellopontine angle. Once the surgical field is selected and set up, the endoscope is placed close to the sigmoid-transverse junction and held in place with the Mitaka Point Setter Pneumatic Holding System (Mitaka Kohki Co Ltd, Tokyo, Japan). As previously described, this is a pneumatically driven and powered holding retractor which uses pressurized nitrogen. Once set in place it does not move which is of paramount importance given the tight working space and critical neural structures present in the field.

Patient Positioning

The patient is placed in a Mayfield type 3 pin cranial clamp to assure no movement of the head during surgery. The patient is placed on a lateral decubitus position with an axillary roll. Care is taken to thoroughly tape the patient to the surgical table with generous amounts of 3 inch tape. The affected side should be up and the shoulder gently taped inferiorly to increase exposure to the area of approach. Only a small amount of hair needs to be clipped behind the ear (Fig. 4). External landmarks can be used to localize the transverse sinus (inion to zygomatic arch line) and sigmoid sinus (medial aspect of

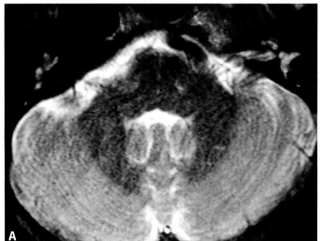 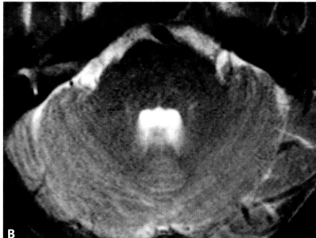

Figs. 3A and B: T_2-weighted axial MRI of patient presenting with left-sided classical trigeminal neuralgia and evidence of a large, ectatic vertebral artery compressing the dorsal root entry zone.

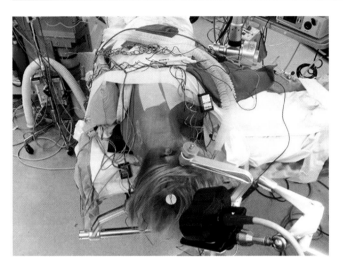

Fig. 4: Positioning of patient for endovascular decompression of left trigeminal nerve. The Mayfield head clamp is used for cranial stabilization. Intraoperative sensory-motor mapping is done. Care is taken to fully secure the patient to the surgical bed to prevent any movement during surgery.

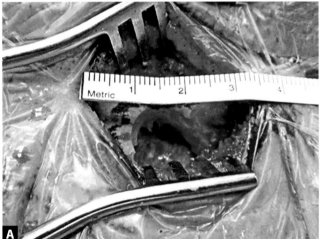

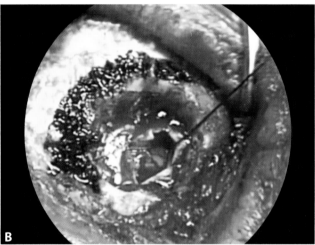

Figs. 5A and B: For an endoscopic only approach, a single burr hole is placed underneath the junction of the transverse sigmoid sinuses. The dura is then opened in a cruciate fashion after obtaining drain relaxation.

mastoid process along the digastric groove). The junction of these two lines will indicate the transverse-sigmoid sinuses junction. However, the use of neuronavigation allows for easy and accurate localization of this important landmark. The surgery is performed under general anesthesia using standard protocols. Neuromonitoring, if available, can be used to help identify the facial nerve and monitor for unwarranted stretch or injury.

Surgical Approach

The scalp is prepped with povidone-iodine solution and allowed to adequately dry for full effect. A single dose of antibiotics is given prior to skin incision. A single linear incision is made with its epicenter over the proposed burr hole site. The monopolar unit, with the needle tip attachment, is set at 20 W and used to incise the dermis

and dissect down to bone. A subperiosteal elevation of the nuchal musculature is also done with the monopolar. It is very important to achieve maximal cerebellar relaxation which may be accomplished in several ways. A combination of mild hyperventilation and diuretics (mannitol ± lasix) can be used. Alternatively, a lumbar drain can be placed prior to positioning the patient and enough CSF can be removed to obtain sufficient relaxation. Neuronavigation is then used (if available) to properly localize the placement of the burr hole which can be made with an electric, pneumatic, or hand drill. The burr hole can be enlarged at the base in order to maximize the opening and increase the angulation of the endoscope (Fig. 5A). Once the dura is exposed, it can be sharply opened in a cruciate fashion (Fig. 5B) and suspended with a suture anteriorly against the sigmoid

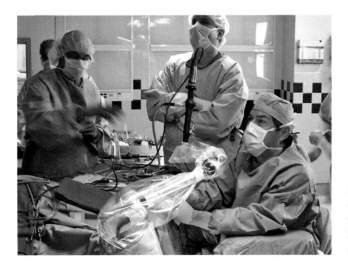

Fig. 6: Operating room set up shows surgeon sitting on an operating room stool equipped with arm rests. Gently resting the arms/elbows on the arm rests decreases surgeon fatigue and increase arm/hand stability. It also allows for usage of feet to control foot pedals for irrigation and/or cautery.

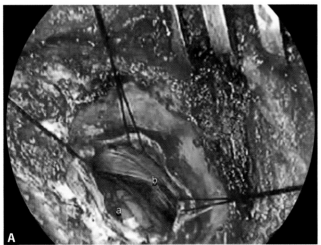
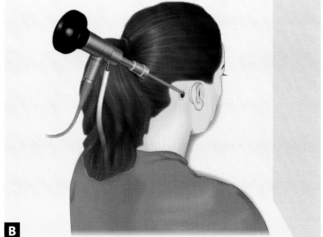

Figs. 7A and B: (A) Surgical view of burr hole and dural opening showing adequate cerebellar decompression. The cerebellum (a) is appropriately retracted from the petrus pyramid (b); (B) Approximate angle of approach used for the endoscopic microvascular decompression of lower cranial nerves.

sinus. As with all other endoscopic procedures, it is the author's preference to sit on an operating room chair with movable arm holders. These holders are set such that the surgeon's elbows can rest comfortably on them at approximately 90° angles. This set up significantly decreases surgeon's fatigability and allows for the use of all limbs (both hands to manipulate surgical instruments and feet for controlling irrigation and bipolar coagulation) (Fig. 6). Given the small opening, the preferred set of endoscopic instruments are the Sephrina by Karl Storz which minimize space conflicts with the endoscope. The diameter of the endoscope may vary from 2.7 mm to 4.0 mm. These can be used interchangeably in order to obtain maximal working space.

Microvascular Decompression

After adequate patient positioning, cerebellar relaxation, and dural opening, the endoscope is carefully guided along the wall of the petrous pyramid (Figs. 7A and B). Care is taken to visualize the tentorium and its junction with the petrous bone. Minimal retraction should be necessary. The cranial nerves should be easily identified as they enter the petrous bone through their respective canals covered with arachnoid membrane (Fig. 8). Micro scissors are used to perform dissection of the arachnoid sheath surrounding the cranial nerves (Fig. 9). A key maneuver is to position the endoscope close enough to get full visualization of the surgical field yet not so

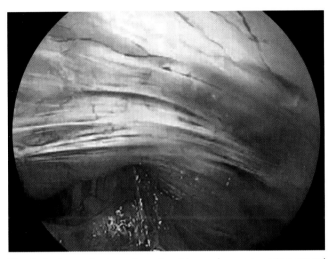

Fig. 8: Endoscopic view of arachnoid membrane covering neural and vascular structures as they enter the petrous bone's canals.

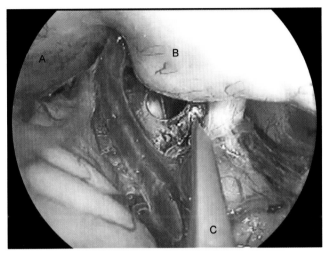

Fig. 9: The cerebellopontine angle is visualized with the tentorium (A) and petrous (B) being seen superiorly. An arachnoid knife (C) is used to carefully dissect the arachnoid over the neurovascular structures.

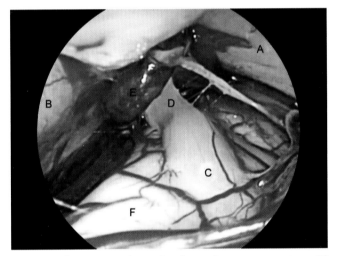

Fig. 10: Close up endoscopic view of venous structure (E) compressing and indenting trigeminal nerve (D) distal to the root entry zone (C) and the pons (F) the tentorium (A) and petrous bones (B) are also visualized.

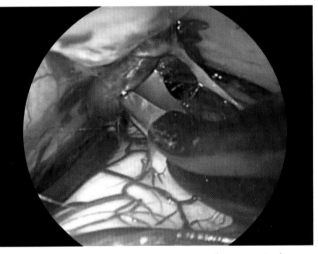

Fig. 11: The venous structure compressing the trigeminal nerve is gently shrunk with bipolar electrocautery and to create space for placing the Teflon pledget.

close as to compromise instrument triangulation. Once the trigeminal nerve has been identified, the endoscope can be rigidly fixated in the Mitaka Point Setter holder and secured in place. Further microsurgical dissection of arachnoid and surrounding vessels is undertaken. At this point the offending vessels can be identified (Fig. 10). Careful manipulation of the neural and vascular structures allow for placement of a Teflon pledget in order to separate the offending vessel from the nerve or its root entry zone (Figs. 11 and 12).

CLINICAL CASES

Case 1

A 47-year-old female presented with classical symptoms of left-sided glossopharyngeal neuralgia. Preoperative MRI workup demonstrated a large and ectatic vertebral artery compressing the brainstem. She was taken to surgery where an endoscopic MVD was successfully performed. At the time of surgery (Fig. 13) a large vertebral artery could be seen compressing critical

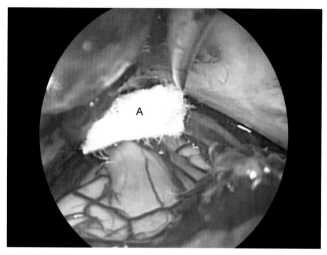

Fig. 12: A Teflon pledget (A) being placed between the trigeminal nerve and compressing vascular structure.

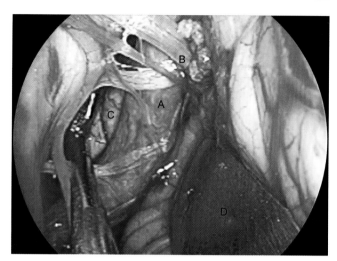

Fig. 13: Endoscopic view of a large, ectatic vertebral artery (A) compressing the exiting lower cranial nerve IX (B) and medulla (C). A small brain retractor (D) gently holds the cerebellar hemisphere.

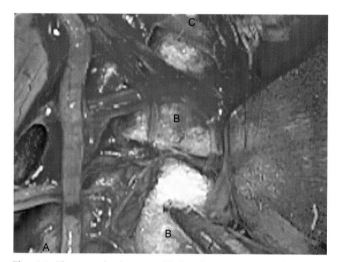

Fig. 14: The vertebral artery (A) has been separated from the cranial nerve rootlets (C) by the Teflon pledgets (B) providing relief of symptoms to the patient.

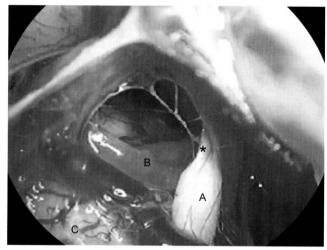

Fig. 15: Surgical view of patient with left-sided trigeminal neuralgia. The exiting CNV (A) can be seen being indented (*) by an arterial vessel loop (B). The Pons (C) is also visualized. (CNV: Trigeminal cranial nerve or the fifth cranial nerve).

neural structures. The patient was successfully decompressed (Fig. 14) and remains symptom-free 5 years postoperative.

Case 2

A 36-year-old male presented to clinic with a 5-year history of classical left-sided TN. MRIs were negative. At surgery, an arterial vessel loop was seen compressing the trigeminal nerve (Figs. 15 and 16). He was decompressed (Fig. 17) and remains symptom-free 7 years postoperative.

Case 3

An otherwise healthy 25-year-old female presented with TN of several years duration. Overall, preoperative workup was negative. At surgery, an arterial vessel was seen pulsating on and indenting the trigeminal nerve's

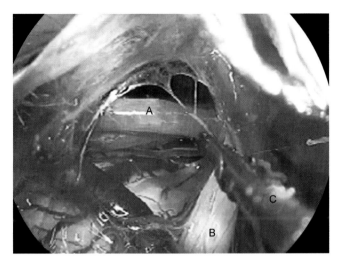

Fig. 16: The arterial vessel loop (A) is being mobilized from the trigeminal nerve (B) with the aid of a microscopic dissector (C).

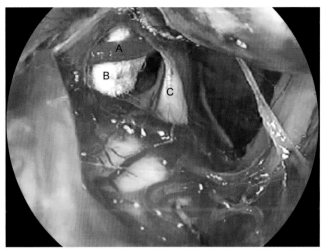

Fig. 17: The vessel loop (A) has been separated from the trigeminal nerve (C) by the pledget of Teflon (B).

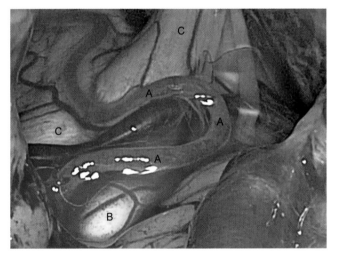

Fig. 18: Endoscopic view of clinical case 3 depicts an arterial vessel loop (A) compressing the patient's trigeminal root entry zone (B and C) and the nerve (C).

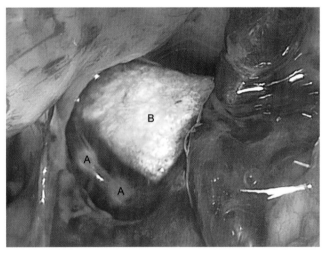

Fig. 19: The vessel loop (A) has been elevated from the trigeminal nerve by the Teflon pledget (B).

root entry zone (Fig. 18). A pledget of Teflon was used to successfully decompress the nerve (Fig. 19).

CLOSURE

Inspection of the endoscopic field should demonstrate adequate decompression of the neural structures. The field is irrigated and filled with normothermic lactated ringers. The dura is closed primarily with neurolon, if possible. If not, a piece of muscle and/or dural substitute can be placed over the dura along with a piece of gelfoam. A single burr hole cover can be used to cover the bony defect and prevent postoperative deformity or pain. Subcutaneous and dermal closure is done in a standard fashion.

COMPLICATIONS

Complications for MVD include hearing loss, trochlear nerve palsy, CSF leakage, intracranial bleeding, and trauma or infarction. Mortality, mainly due to cerebellar/ brain stem infarction, ranges between 0.2% and 1.2%.[30] The incidences of hearing impairment and cerebral injury have decreased since the early 1990s due to the institution of BSER (brainstem evoked response) monitoring during surgery.[3,31] General advancements in surgical technique have also aided in the improvement of patient outcomes.

CONCLUSION

Microvascular decompression is capable of safely curing TN due to vascular compression. By approaching the operation endoscopically, surgeons can enhance visualization and locate sites of neurovascular conflict with greater ease. Because endoscopic surgery is more thorough and less invasive than traditional methods, the patient has a better chance of achieving an immediate, pain-free postoperative period as well as a shorter recovery. Generally speaking, patients with typical presentation and severe arterial compression seem to have a better chance at achieving a successful surgical outcome and avoiding TN recurrence.

REFERENCES

1. Chen MJ, Zhang WJ, Yang C, et al. Endoscopic neurovascular perspective in microvascular decompression of trigeminal neuralgia. J Craniomaxillofac Surg. 2008;36(8):456-61.
2. Katusic S, Beard CM, Bergstralh E, et al. Incidence and clinical features of trigeminal neuralgia, Rochester, Minnesota, 1945-1984. Ann Neurol. 1990;27(1):89-95.
3. Chung SS. Microvascular decompression for trigeminal neuralgia. In: Lozano A, Gildenberg P, Tasker R (Eds). Textbook of Stereotactic and Functional Neurosurgery. Berlin Heidelberg: Springer; 2009. pp. 2465-74.
4. Gardner WJ. Concerning the mechanism of trigeminal neuralgia and hemifacial spasm. J Neurosurg. 1962;19:947-58.
5. Kerr FW. Pathology of trigeminal neuralgia: light and electron microscopic observations. J Neurosurg. 1967;26(1 Suppl):151-6.
6. Sindou M, Howeidy T, Acevedo G. Anatomical observations during microvascular decompression for idiopathic trigeminal neuralgia (with correlations between topography of pain and site of the neurovascular conflict). Prospective study in a series of 579 patients. Acta Neurochir (Wien). 2002;144(1):1-12; discussion 12-3.
7. Setty P, Volkov AA, D'Andrea KP, et al. Endoscopic vascular decompression for the treatment of trigeminal neuralgia: clinical outcomes and technical note. World Neurosurg. 2014;81(3-4):603-8.
8. Cai Q, Song P, Chen Q, et al. Neuroendoscopic fenestration of the septum pellucidum for monoventricular hydrocephalus. Clin Neurol Neurosurg. 2013;115(7):976-80.
9. El-Garem HF, Badr-El-Dine M, Talaat AM, et al. Endoscopy as a tool in minimally invasive trigeminal neuralgia surgery. Otol Neurotol. 2002;23(2):132-5.
10. Jarrahy R, Berci G, Shahinian HK. Endoscope-assisted microvascular decompression of the trigeminal nerve. Otolaryngol—Head Neck Surg. 2000;123(3):218-23.
11. Sandell T, Ringstad GA, Eide PK. Usefulness of the endoscope in microvascular decompression for trigeminal neuralgia and MRI-based prediction of the need for endoscopy. Acta Neurochir (Wien). 2014;156(10):1901-9.
12. Rak R, Sekhar LN, Stimac D, et al. Endoscope-assisted microsurgery for microvascular compression syndromes. Neurosurgery. 2004;54(4):876-81; discussion 881-3.
13. Jarrahy R, Eby JB, Cha ST, et al. Fully endoscopic vascular decompression of the trigeminal nerve. Minim Invas Neurosurg. 2002;45(1):32-5.
14. Lee A, McCartney S, Burbidge C, et al. Trigeminal neuralgia occurs and recurs in the absence of neurovascular compression. J Neurosurg. 2014;120(5):1048-54.
15. Pagura JR. Microvascular decompression for trigeminal neuralgia. In: Lozano A, Gildenberg P, Tasker R (Eds). Textbook of Stereotactic and Functional Neurosurgery. Berlin Heidelberg: Springer; 2009. pp. 1911-23.
16. Cheng J, Lei D, Zhang H, et al. Trigeminal root compression for trigeminal neuralgia in patients with no vascular compression. Acta Neurochir. 2015;157(2):323-7.
17. Young JN, Wilkins RH. Partial sensory trigeminal rhizotomy at the pons for trigeminal neuralgia. J Neurosurg. 1993;79(5):680-7.
18. Zakrzewska JM, Lopez BC, Kim SE, et al. Patient reports of satisfaction after microvascular decompression and partial sensory rhizotomy for trigeminal neuralgia. Neurosurgery. 2005;56(6):1304-11; discussion 1311-2.
19. Teo C, Nakaji P, Mobbs RJ. Endoscope-assisted microvascular decompression for trigeminal neuralgia: technical case report. Neurosurgery. 2006;59(4 Suppl 2):ONSE489-90.
20. Barker FG 2nd, Jannetta PJ, Bissonette DJ, et al. The long-term outcome of microvascular decompression for trigeminal neuralgia. N Engl J Med. 1996;334(17):1077-83.
21. Kabil MS, Eby JB, Shahinian HK. Endoscopic vascular decompression versus microvascular decompression of the trigeminal nerve. Minim Invas Neurosurg. 2005;48(4):207-12.
22. Burchiel KJ, Clarke H, Haglund M, et al. Long-term efficacy of microvascular decompression in trigeminal neuralgia. J Neurosurg. 1988;69(1):35-8.
23. Li ST, Pan Q, Liu N, et al. Trigeminal neuralgia: what are the important factors for good operative outcomes with

microvascular decompression. Surg Neurol. 2004;62(5):400-4; discussion 404-5.

24. Miller JP, Magill ST, Acar F, et al. Predictors of long-term success after microvascular decompression for trigeminal neuralgia. J Neurosurg. 2009;110(4):620-6.

25. Sindou M, Leston J, Decullier E, et al. Microvascular decompression for primary trigeminal neuralgia: long-term effectiveness and prognostic factors in a series of 362 consecutive patients with clear-cut neurovascular conflicts who underwent pure decompression. J Neurosurg. 2007;107(6):1144-53.

26. Sun T, Saito S, Nakai O, et al. Long-term results of microvascular decompression for trigeminal neuralgia with reference to probability of recurrence. Acta Neurochir. 1994;126(2-4):144-8.

27. Dahle L, von Essen C, Kourtopoulos H, et al. Microvascular decompression for trigeminal neuralgia. Acta Neurochir. 1989;99(3-4):109-12.

28. Tyler-Kabara EC, Kassam AB, Horowitz MH, et al. Predictors of outcome in surgically managed patients with typical and atypical trigeminal neuralgia: comparison of results following microvascular decompression. J Neurosurg. 2002;96(3):527-31.

29. Gu W, Zhao W. Microvascular decompression for recurrent trigeminal neuralgia. J Clin Neurosci. 2014;21(9):1549-53.

30. Sindou M. Microvascular decompression for trigeminal neuralgia. In: Sindou M (Ed). Practical Handbook of Neurosurgery. Vienna: Springer; 2009. pp. 1448-62.

31. McLaughlin MR, Jannetta PJ, Clyde BL, et al. Microvascular decompression of cranial nerves: lessons learned after 4400 operations. J Neurosurg. 1999;90(1):1-8.

CHAPTER 14

Endoscopic Carpal Tunnel Release

David F Jimenez, Michael J McGinity

INTRODUCTION

Median nerve compression in the carpal tunnel was described by Sir James Paget in 1853, but it was not until 1933 that Learmonth first described a surgical procedure to release the compressed nerve at the wrist. First popularized by Phalen, a surgeon at the Mayo Clinic in the 1950s, open and direct transection of the transverse carpal ligament has become the standard surgical technique for the surgical treatment carpal tunnel syndrome. Multiple variations of the open technique have been described over the years by various surgeons. Okutsu, a Japanese orthopaedic surgeon, in 1986 was the first to perform and report on the release of the transverse carpal ligament (TLC) in patients with carpal tunnel syndrome using an endoscopic technique. Since the introduction of endoscopic carpal tunnel release, several authors have championed different endoscopic techniques in order to release the entrapped median nerve. Endoscopic procedures are generally divided into two categories based on the number of incisions made to introduce the endoscopic instrumentation. Single portal techniques include those developed by Okutsu, Menon, and Agee. Double portal techniques include procedures introduced by Chow, Resnick and Miller and lastly Brown. Presented in this chapter is the two-portal technique as described by Brown. This technique is described in detail because the senior author has found it to be the most reliable, safe and efficacious of all of the endoscopic techniques.

PATIENT SELECTION

Endoscopic release of the TCL should be reserved for those patients with classical signs and symptoms of idiopathic carpal tunnel syndrome. This category accounts for ~43% of carpal tunnel syndrome cases. Symptoms may include a dull ache and pain or discomfort of the hand, forearm, or upper arm, hand paresthesias, weakness of the hand, and nocturnal paresthesias relieved with shaking of the hand. Provocative factors inducing these findings include sustained hand or arm position and repetitive action of the hand or wrist. Physical examination may be normal, but many patients present with positive Phalen's or Tinel's sign, thenar musculature weakness and/or atrophy, and sensory loss in the distribution of the median nerve. The patient who fails to improve following an adequate trial of conservative therapy and has positive electrodiagnostic studies becomes a candidate for endoscopic release of TCL. Systemic cause of carpal tunnel syndrome, such as acromegaly, thyroid disease, pregnancy, and proliferative tenosynovitis, must be ruled out before considering endoscopic carpal tunnel release. Several conditions preclude dissection of the TCL with the endoscopic technique. Contraindications include a history of open carpal tunnel release and patients with proliferative tenosynovitis or concomitant ulnar nerve entrapment. Patients with mass lesions (e.g. neuromas) should not undergo endoscopic operation. Patients with a history of previous trauma or anatomical anomalies should be excluded as well.

PREOPERATIVE PREPARATION

Anesthetic management of patients undergoing endoscopic carpal tunnel release can be either local, regional, or general. Many surgeons advocate the use of local or regional anesthesia (Bier block). However, the authors'

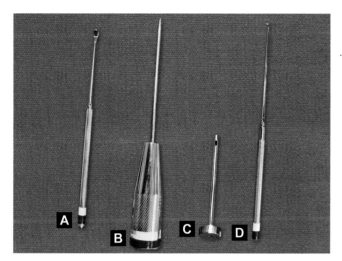

Fig. 1: Endotrac endoscopic instruments used for carpal tunnel release: (A) synovial elevator, (B) obturator, (C) slotted cannula, (D) right angle probe.

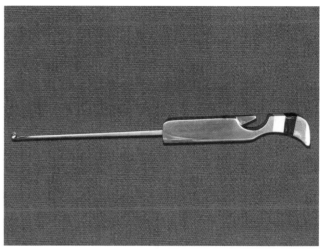

Fig. 2: Handle with disposable hook blade used for transecting the transverse carpal ligament.

preferred method is rapid mask general anesthesia. This is quickly and easily done using propofol and does not require endotracheal intubation. Following placement of an intravenous line, a bolus of propofol is given at 1 mg/kg followed by continuous infusion of 100 mg/kg/h. Induction is immediate, as is its reversal. Generally, the procedure lasts between 5 minutes and 10 minutes. Using this method, the patient is totally pain-free during the procedure and amnestic for the event. Patients are discharged 1–2 hours following the procedure and full recovery from anesthesia. However, patients with history of esophageal reflux or with other complicating factors should be operated upon using regional or endotracheal general anesthesia.

OPERATIVE PROCEDURE

Positioning

With the patient in the supine position, the affected arm is placed extended on a hand table or an arm board, and a tourniquet is placed above the elbow. The hand and forearm are prepped with povidone–iodine scrub and paint followed by standard draping and impermeable and split sheets. It is very important that the surgeon's dominant hand be situated closest to the patient and this will vary with patient's affected hand and side of surgeon's dominance. The television monitors should be placed directly across from the surgeon as well as the assistant.

Instrumentation

The equipment necessary to perform this procedure is found in all modern hospitals: television monitors, a rigid 4-mm, 30° endoscope or arthroscopes with light source, and mounted camera. The specific endoscopic instruments (Endotrac™ system) (Fig. 1) are manufactured by Instratek (Houston, TX) and consist of ergonomically well-designed obturator-cannula complex for entering the carpal tunnel and disposable hook knife (Fig. 2). Although the equipment is sold as a set or separately, the entire procedure can be performed with only three instruments: (1) a synovial elevator, (2) an obturator, and (3) a hook knife. Other instruments available include raspers, probes, and retractors. The synovial elevator is used to ascertain the appropriate plane of dissection as well as to remove synovium from the undersurface of the TCL. The obturator consists of a rigid 4-mm tapered rod encased in a removable slotted cannula. Once inserted, the open end of the cannula should lie against the undersurface of the TCL. Following insertion of the endoscope, the 30° angle lens will afford an excellent view of the TCL. There are several types of blades and knives available to section the ligament. Manufacturers make hook, forward, and triangular blades. The only other instruments needed to perform this procedure are a ruler, a marking pen, a single-toothed Adson's forceps (Codman, Raynham, Massachusetts), and tenotomy scissors.

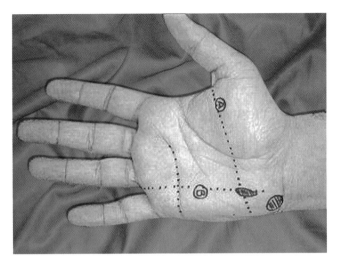

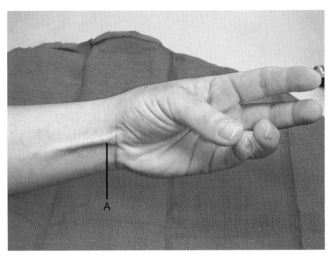

Fig. 3: Kaplan's cardinal line (A) is a line parallel to the the extended base of the first digit. A parallel line to the ulnar aspect of the ring finger (B) crosses Kaplan's line at the level of the hook of the hamate.

Fig. 4: The tendon of the palmaris longus (A) is localized in the distal forearm by asking the patient to flex the wrist and opose the thumb and the 5th digit. The incision is made immediately ulnar to this tendon.

Anatomical Landmarks

Complete familiarity with anatomical landmarks of the median nerve and associated structures of the carpal tunnel is essential for a safe and excellent outcome. Several superficial landmarks can assist the surgeon and adequately plan the surgical approach. Kaplan's cardinal line extends along the base of the extended thumb and runs parallel to the distal palmar crease. A line can be drawn perpendicular to the distal wrist crease and located along the ulnar side of the fourth digit. The intersection of these two lines indicates the location of the hook of the hamate, or the most ulnar extent of the TCL. Kaplan's line approximates the most distant edge of the TCL, which blends proximally, at the distal wrist crease with an antebrachial fascia (Fig. 3). The median nerve is located on the radial aspect of the carpal tunnel and radial to the palmaris longus tendon. The ulnar nerve enters the palm on the ulnar aspect of the hook of the hamate and into the Guyon's canal. The palmar arterial arch is located 1 cm to 2 cm distal to the edge of the TCL. Therefore, there exists a small anatomical corridor devoid of major neurovascular structures, where the TCL can be safely sectioned using endoscopic techniques.

Procedure

Prior to anesthetic induction, the video equipment is connected and checked for proper functioning. The camera should be white-balanced and the appropriate orientation should be obtained so that the TV monitor image correlates with the appropriate patient spatial orientation. The skin landmarks are ascertained at this point. The patient is asked to flex the wrist and oppose the thumb and fifth digit to visualize the palmaris longus tendon (if present). The distal wrist crease is the most important landmark because all others are based on its location. The proximal port (incision) is placed in an area located between 1 cm and 2 cm proximal to the distal wrist crease. The incision is placed immediately ulnar to the palmaris longus tendon (Fig. 4) (if absent, use the thenar crease as a landmark instead). Often, the incision can be made in the proximal wrist crease and the incision should measure 1 cm or less. Next, a point is marked 3 cm distal to the distal wrist crease in a link directed toward the third webspace. In the majority of patients, this will mark the end of the distal TCL ± 0.25 cm. Along the same line, a dot is marked at 4 cm distal to the wrist crease and a 0.5 cm circle is drawn circumferentially (Fig. 5).

This circle encompasses the safe area where the distal stab incision can be made. The corridor between the proximal and distal portals encompasses the area where only the TCL is present and well-visualized. The median nerve, located radial to the palmaris longus tendon, is outside this corridor as well as the palmar arch, which is located distal to the 4 cm circle and the ulnar nerve, which is located lateral to the hook of the hamate. The

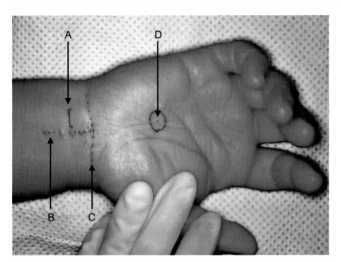

Fig. 5: Landmarks used for endoscopic release of the transverse carpal ligament. The carpal tunnel is accessed via a small incision (A) located immediately ulnar to palmaris longus tendon (B) and proximal to the distal wrist crease (C). The exit site (D) is 4 cm distal to (C) along the third webspace.

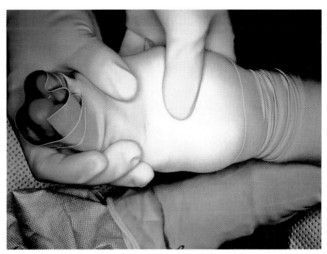

Fig. 6: The hand and forearm are exsanguinated using an Esmarch rubber band and the tourniquet is inflated to 250 mm Hg.

superficial sensory branches of the ulnar and median nerves as well as the recurrent motor branch of the median nerve lie well outside this corridor. As previously mentioned, familiarity with external landmarks is important to understand the underlying anatomy. A line is drawn perpendicular to the distal crease along the ulnar aspect of the fourth digit. A second line, Kaplan's cardinal line, which extends along the first webspace and parallel to the distal palmar crease, is also marked. The intersection of these lines marks the location of the hamate. The distal border of the TCL lies in close proximity to Kaplan's line.

Following induction, the arm is elevated and a rubber Esmarch bandage (Trinity Laboratories, Inc., Salisbury, Maryland) is applied to exsanguinate the extremity (Fig. 6). The tourniquet is inflated to pressures above systolic, and the Esmarch bandage is removed. The hand is placed in slight extension on a pair of towels. The proximal incision is made immediately ulnar to the palmaris longus with a no. 15 blade, taking care not to extend more than 1 cm in the ulnar direction (Fig. 7). Once the dermis is cut, tenotomy scissors are used to spread the subcutaneous tissue apart and allow visualization of the volar antebrachial fascial fibers (Fig. 8). Following exposure, the fibers are spread apart with the scissor tips, thereby gaining entrance into the carpal tunnel. At this point, the longitudinally running tendons may be easily visualized. Adson's forceps are

used to grasp and elevate the distal edge of the divided antebrachial fascia. The synovial elevator is then gently inserted under the fascial fibers and advanced distally at an acute angle (40° to 60°) (Fig. 9). Once the tip of the elevator advances past the distal wrist crease, it is angled superiorly to feel the undersurface of the transversely running fibers. This anatomical orientation will produce a "washboard"-type sensation as the tip of the elevator moves across the transverse fibers. Further advancement of the elevator into the palm will allow the surgeon to kinesthetically feel the distal border of the TCL. This edge will be identified by the lack of washboard feel and soft passage into the palm's fat pad.

Prior to removal of the elevator, the antebrachial fascia should be grasped to maintain an open tract into the carpal tunnel. Next, an obturator-cannula assembly is inserted into the tract beneath the TCL. As the obturator is passed distally into the tunnel, the hand and wrist should be maintained in a neutral position. Ulnar pressure should be applied to the obturator to maintain the tip immediately radial to the hook of the hamate. This maneuver will ensure that Guyon's canal is not entered. Once the obturator tip is passed beyond the hook of the hamate, the wrist is extended to 30°. As the distal edge of the TCL is passed, the surgeon's nondominant hand is used to apply pressure over the 4 cm marked circle. The tip of the obturator should be easily felt under the palmar skin. Ventral pressure is applied as the tip of the obturator is pushed dorsally. At this point, only skin lies between the surgeon's thumb and the obturator's tip. A

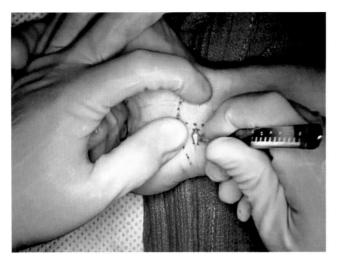

Fig. 7: A scalpel is used to incise the skin and expose the antebrachial fascia.

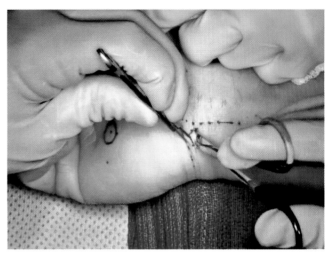

Fig. 8: The antebrachial fascia is longitudinally dissected using a pair of tenotomy scissors.

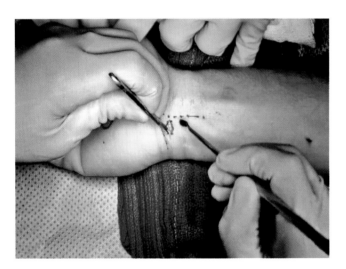

Fig. 9: A synovial elevator is placed under the antebrachial fascia and advanced into the carpal tunnel.

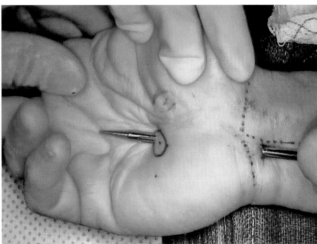

Fig. 10: An obturator with a slotted cannula is inserted into the proximal incision, placed incised the carpal tunnel and exits 4 cm distal along the third webspace.

small stab wound is made over the obturator's tip and should be visualized with slight forward pressure. The obturator-cannula assembly is then pushed through the distal portal (Fig. 10). The obturator is removed and the cannula is left in the palm aligned with the open side facing superiorly (Fig. 11). The open ended terminus of the cannula will extend from the palmar incision to allow the endoscope to be inserted (Fig. 12). A 30°, upward facing angled endoscope is used to visualize the undersurface of the TCL (Fig. 13). The tip of the lighted endoscope is inserted into the distal end of the cannula (Fig. 14). A disposable hook blade is used to transect the TCL

(Fig. 15). The assistant then inserts the rigid scope into the distal end of the cannula. Proximal advancement of the scope will allow full visualization of the entire undersurface of the TCL. White, glistening, transversely oriented fibers should be visualized (Fig. 16). The surgeon inserts the hook blade assembly into the proximal port of the cannula and, as the blade moves, the assistant moves the scope in the same direction maintaining a separation of several millimeters. The blade is moved toward the distal end of the TCL where the palmar fat pad is visualized. The edge of the ligament is then hooked with the hook blade, and with a steady, strong, proximal pull the TCL

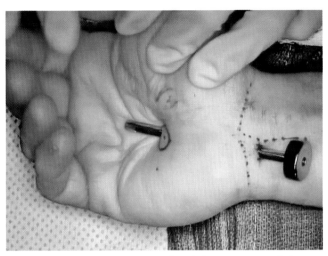

Fig. 11: The obturator is removed and the open cannula is rotated 15° ulnarward.

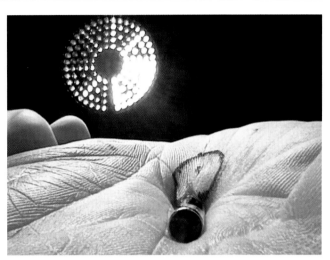

Fig. 12: Endoscopic view of distal end of cannula exiting out the distal incision. The open side of the cannula is in direct contact with the undersurface of the transverse carpal ligament.

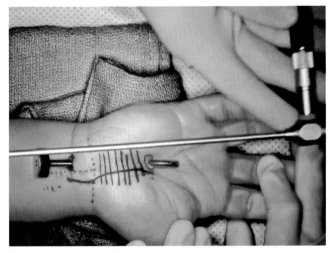

Fig. 13: An angled 30° endoscope is used to visualize the undersurface of the transverse carpal ligament. The angled end of the endoscope is aimed superiorly as seen in this photograph.

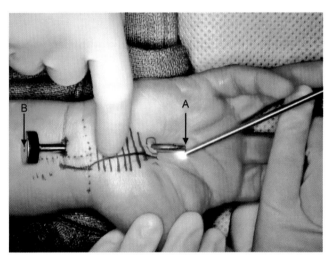

Fig. 14: The endoscope is inserted into the distal end of the cannula (A) at the palm. The hook blade is inserted, using the surgeon's dominant hand, with the proximal end of the cannula (B).

is divided (Figs. 17 and 18). As soon as the full thickness of the ligament is cut, the overlying palmar fat pad will fall into view and commonly obstructs the view through the endoscope. The scope is moved back and forth and, if ligament sections have not been divided, a second or third pass may be necessary to complete full sectioning. A full-thickness cut can be ascertained by rotating the cannula and directly visualizing the cut ends of the TCL's fibers on either side. The principle is to insert the working channel inside the ulnar aspect of the carpal tunnel. Only the offending agent (the TCL) is cut. Other normal structures such as the skin, the fat pad, and the palmaris

brevis tendon are left intact. With the entire ligament is inspected and sectioned, the endoscope and cannula are removed. Care must be taken not to cut or fully section a flexor tendon (Fig. 19). Anytime longitudinally running fibers are seen coursing in a proximal-distal direction. A tendon must be suspected, in such case the fingers must be flexed and extended forcefully to see if these fibers move back and forth in a proximial-distal direction. If such is the case, the obturator is reinserted in the cannula, both are removed from the carpal tunnel and a new pass is attempted. Once the ligament is fully transected, the palmar fat pad falls into the endoscopic surgical field

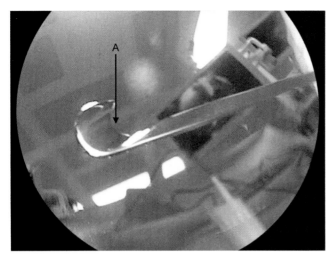

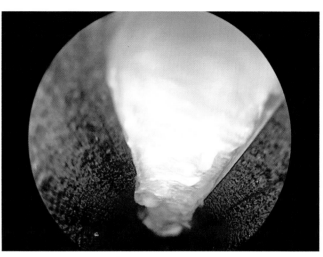

Fig. 15: A disposable hook blade is used to cut the transverse carpal ligament. The cutting edge (A) is moved in a distal to proximal direction. Several passes may be needed with very thick and brittle ligaments.

Fig. 16: The proper endoscopic view shows the undersurface of transverse carpal ligament with its white, shiny fibers running transversely across the field. A small amount of synovium is seen on the edges of the cannula.

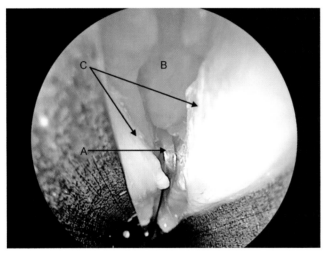

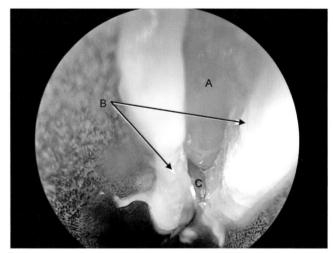

Fig. 17: The hook blade (A) is seen cutting the transverse carpal ligament and its sectioned edges (C) are easily visualized as well as the palmar fat pad (B) above the TCL. (TCL: Transverse carpal ligament).

Fig. 18: Another patient shows the blade (C) cutting the transverse carpal ligament and its sectioned edges (B) as well as the palmar fat pad (A).

(Fig. 20) obscuring the rest of the anatomical landmarks. This indicates complete and successful TCL sectioning. The tourniquet is deflated and any bleeding is controlled with pressure (2–5 minutes) (Fig. 21) and/or bipolar electrocautery. The skin is closed with subcuticular 4-0 Monocryl and the skin sealed within dermabond (Fig. 22). No dressing, splint, or sling are used. The patient is allowed to resume unrestricted activities within the limits of comfort. Several weeks following surgery typically demonstrate superb healing and minimal scarring.

To procure the best possible results with two-portal endoscopic release of the TCL, the following check points should be recognized: (1) The "washboard" sensation must be felt with the tip of the synovial elevator and obturator. If this does not occur, the obturator may be above the TCL. (2) The whitish, transversely oriented fibers of the TCL must be clearly visualized. Longitudinally running fibers may be indicative of a tendon or the median nerve. (3) The edges of the sectioned TCL must be clearly visualized bilaterally along the entire length of the ligament.

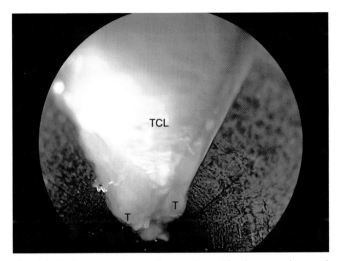

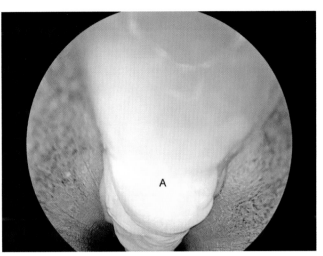

Fig. 19: Endoscopic views of cannula inside the carpal tunnel. The metal cannula extends from about 1 o'clock to 11 o'clock. The superior aspect exposes the undersurface of the transverse carpal ligament whose white, glistening fibers run transversely across the field. Flexor tendons (T) can be seen running longitudinally along the cannula's axis. (TCL: Transverse carpal ligament).

Fig. 20: Once the transverse carpal ligament has been fully transected, the palmar fat pad (A) falls through the cut ligament and completely fills the field of view, indicating complete release of the carpal tunnel.

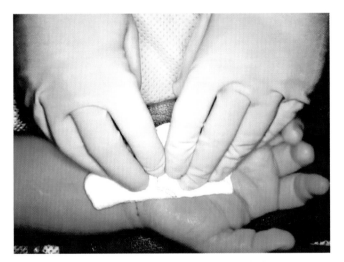

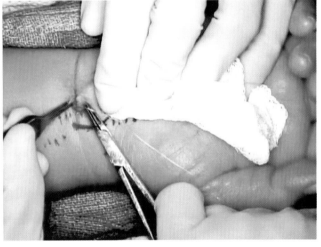

Fig. 21: After the instruments are removed and the tourniquet is deflated, pressure is applied for approximately 5 minutes to minimize the risk of postoperative hematoma.

Fig. 22: The incisions are closed using 4.0 Monocryl for the subcuticular layer and dermabond for the skin. No bandages, splints or slings are used postoperatively and the patient is encouraged to begin using the hand early on.

Failure to observe these checkpoints will place the patient at risk for a complication or poor result.

POSTOPERATIVE MANAGEMENT, INCLUDING POSSIBLE COMPLICATIONS

Resolution of symptoms in 98% of the patients can be expected with this procedure. The overall complication rate was 0.9% with one flexor tendon laceration. Reflex sympathetic dystrophy developed in 0.4% of patients.

Overall, there was a 2% recurrence rate. The patients in this group returned to work after an average of 15 days. Complications associated with other endoscopic tunnel release approaches are not insignificant. These include median nerve transection, superficial palmar arch injury, flexor tendon lacerations, ulnar nerve transection, pseudoaneurysm formation in the palmar arch, reflex sympathetic dystrophy, transient neurapraxias, and paresthesias as well as incomplete release of the TCL.

CONCLUSION

With the development of endoscopic techniques and new instruments for the release of carpal tunnel syndrome, surgeons as well as patients are provided with alternate measures and treatment choices. Results with the biportal endoscopic carpal tunnel release compare favorably with the standard open technique. There is significantly less pillar pain, less scarring, and rapid return of pinch grip strength with early return to work times. The operation can usually be performed within 10 minutes, with an average tourniquet time of less than 5 minutes. Careful patient selection and adherence to the surgical principles described herein should produce excellent results.

CHAPTER 15

Intraventricular Cysts

David F Jimenez, David N Garza

INTRODUCTION

There are primarily three types of cysts that can be found within the ventricular system: (1) choroid plexus cysts (CPCs), (2) ependymal cysts, (3) and colloid cysts.[1] Colloid cysts of the third ventricle have a fibrous external membrane and an inner layer of cuboidal or columnar epithelium (sometimes stratified, often ciliated) which contain mucoid material and epithelial debris.[2] Immunohistochemical studies performed on colloid cyst cells demonstrate the expression of epithelial markers, including cytokeratins and epithelial membrane antigen.[3] As a result of these findings, it has been suggested that colloid cysts have an endodermal origin.[4] This characteristic (hypothetically) distinguishes colloid cysts from CPCs and ependymal cysts, which are both thought to be derived from the primitive neuroepithelium that lines the neural tube. A detailed examination of intraventricular neuroepithelial cysts, specifically CPCs and ependymal cysts, will form the bulk of this report.

The term "neuroepithelial cyst" was first used by Fulton and Bailey in 1920.[3] The designation was originally more broad in application, but it is currently used to describe cysts that develop during embryogenesis within any part of the ventricular system that is lined by neuroepithelium, either by invagination (with a connective tissue layer on the inside of the neuroepithelial layer) or evagination (with the connective tissue on the outside of the neuroepithelial layer).[5] Most neuroepithelial cysts seem to arise from the choroid plexus or ependyma along the anterior portion of the third ventricle adjacent to the foramen of Monro.[6] When the folded epithelium at the site of invagination or evagination is pinched off, tubules form; the obstruction of these tubules and subsequent accumulation of secretory and breakdown products in conjunction with cellular proliferation eventually results in the formation of cysts.[5] Because this process is somewhat gradual, neuroepithelial cysts are most often seen in older patients.[6] Their contents usually include a proteinaceous fluid consisting of cerebrospinal fluid (CSF), lipids, and material reactive to mucicarmine and periodic acid-Schiff stains.[6]

In addition to CPCs and ependymal cysts, arachnoid cysts are also occasionally found within the ventricles, but they have a controversial history that will be discussed later in more detail. Some authors have suggested that arachnoid cysts share several characteristics with neuroepithelial cysts and should be classified as such; others have cited histological and pathophysiological evidence indicating that they are distinct and require their own separate designation. This disparity is only one example of the inconsistent nomenclature associated with intraventricular cyst classification. Although some changes in naming convention can certainly be attributed to advances made in histological and imaging studies, the ongoing diversity of opinion more likely reflects the lack of substantive clinical evidence created by the sheer symptomatic rarity of these cysts. The nomenclature surrounding intracranial epithelial cysts is varied and can be, at times, confusing. For several authors, "colloid cyst" was once considered synonymous with "neuroepithelial cyst".[7] Macgregor et al. used the term "colloid cyst" to describe a cyst related to the ependymal-lined cavities of the brain and spinal cord.[8] Zehnder reported a large subarachnoid cyst arising from the right lateral fissure that was interpreted by different authors as a colloid cyst in 1938, an arachnoid cyst in 1958, and a neuroepithelial cyst in 1975.[9] In the late 1970s, Friede and Yasargil asserted that intracerebral ependymal cysts were distinguishable from intraventricular colloid cysts, but Shuangshoti reported that both cysts are really the same type of lesion.[9] In 1990, Odake et al. combined histologically distinct cysts into a single entity under the general name of "choroid plexus cyst," due to the anatomical location of their attachment in the lateral ventricle.[10,11] This pervasive variation in classification can make it very difficult for researchers who are trying to study intraventricular cysts and accurately distinguish them from each other. Generally speaking, authors use imaging and histochemistry to classify cysts. However, these methods are not always reliable. Cystic contents can appear ambiguous on certain scans, microscopic studies have demonstrated that cyst walls can look different under separate circumstances, and cyst epithelium with multiple cell types can result in immunoreactivity tests that are unclear or inconclusive.[11-13] Additionally, while there are probable theories regarding the precise origin of some of these congenital cysts, definitive explanations for every cyst type have still not fully been elucidated. For all these reasons, regardless of what names they might use for classification purposes, it is of prime importance that the authors who are reporting cyst cases provide as much information as possible when describing their findings. Doing so will assist readers who are trying to compare their work and determine if their comprehension of a given study is accurate.

CHOROID PLEXUS CYSTS

Choroid plexus cysts were first described in a report issued by Chudleigh et al. in 1984 in which they were characterized as benign anatomical variants.[14,15] Most CPCs are bilateral, small (typically measuring 2–8 mm in diameter), and located in the lateral ventricular atria.[1] These cysts tend to concentrate at or around the trigone; congenital cysts localized in the anterior part of the lateral ventricles are very rare.[10] CPCs that are less than 1 cm in diameter are common and seldom symptomatic.[16] They are often detected during routine ultrasonographic studies. If CPCs persist into adulthood, they usually remain silent. Authors have reported incidentally finding them in about 30% of routine autopsy cases.[17] Cysts with a diameter greater than 2 cm are relatively rare but have a greater chance of becoming obstructive and causing hydrocephalic symptoms.[1] Patients with symptomatic CPCs might experience headaches, head enlargement, nausea, vomiting, gait disturbance, and focal epilepsy

(presumably due to direct parenchymal compression).[18,19] Headaches are the most commonly reported symptom; they are often episodic, which is likely due to intermittent obstruction created by dynamic cyst behavior.[18,19] CPCs are usually attached to the choroid plexus, but they can float freely within the ventricle and periodically block normal CSF circulation[18] (Figs. 1A and B). Dynamic cyst behavior has been observed ultrasonographically for many years, but Azab et al. reported what was likely the first intraoperative account of this activity. In 2015, they observed a CPC of the third ventricle intermittently herniate into the lateral ventricle and recede back through the foramen of Monro.[19] CPCs arise when lipids from degenerating and/ or desquamating choroid epithelium accumulate in the choroid plexus.[1] After the plexus becomes lobulated and develops secretory epithelium (primary villi), the rapidly growing choroid plexus gives rise to cysts through the entanglement of villi and subsequent entrapment of CSF.[14] Although histological observations of choroid cyst walls have been somewhat varied within the literature, there are several recurring elements. In 1979, Giorgi reported a symptomatic cyst comprised of a single layer of cuboidal cells that faced the lumen and rested on a thin, loose net of connective tissue.[20] Dempsey and Chandler reported a neoplasm with cyst walls composed of a thin, fibrous membrane lined with low columnar epithelium and no evidence of glial elements.[21] Parizek et al. described a collagenic connective tissue that was covered with basal lamina without epithelial cells.[10] Hatashita encountered a cyst wall that was composed of a thin, loose network of connective tissue, the inner surface of which was lined in part by a single layer of flattened epithelial cells with poorly defined borders.[18]

Choroid plexus cysts are difficult to identify using computed tomographic (CT) or magnetic resonance imaging (MRI) because they have thin, nonenhancing walls and their contents are isodense to CSF.[17] They can only suggest their presence via asymmetric ventriculomegaly (if the foramen of Monro is obstructed) or triventricular hydrocephalus (if they are present in the third ventricle).[17] More specialized MRI sequences, such as FIESTA or 3D CISS, can be used to help define cyst membranes.[22] In a case reported by Filardi et al., it was necessary to implement an additional 3D CISS MR imaging sequence in order to identify an obstructive CPC in the third ventricle and establish a correct diagnosis.[16] With regard to immunohistochemical studies, CPC epithelium (much like normal choroid plexus epithelium) will demonstrate

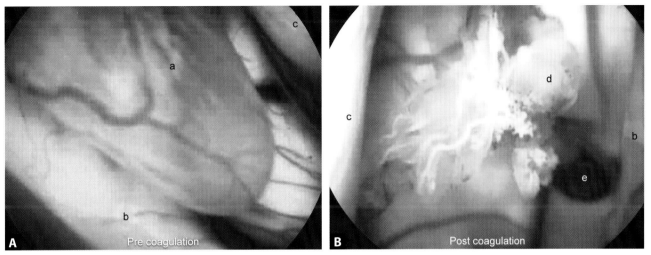

Figs. 1A and B: (A) A 3-year-old presented with intermittent positional headaches secondary to a choroid plexus cyst (a) located near foramen of Monro (e) and between septum pellucidum (b) and the head of the caudate (c). (B) An endoscopic fulguration and shrinkage of the cyst (d) the foramen of Monro (e) was reopened and the patient became asymptomatic.

a strong reactivity for prealbumin (transthyretin), S-100 protein, and cytokeratins.[4,23] CPC epithelium will likely test negative for glial fibrillary acidic protein (GFAP), but some authors have also demonstrated a tendency for choroid plexus papillomas to test positive for GFAP.[3,4,12,13,24] Because of this potential variation in GFAP expression, it might be helpful to test immunoreactivity for prealbumin and S-100 protein in addition to GFAP when trying to diagnosis a lesion: reports have indicated that colloid and enterogenous cysts test negative for all three of those antigens.[4]

The aim of treatment for symptomatic CPCs is to reestablish CSF flow. Several approaches to surgery have been reported, including: simple cyst fenestration, ventriculocystoperitoneal shunting, stereotactic puncture and evacuation, and excision of the cyst wall through various transcortical/transcallosal routes.[10,19,21,25-27] Surgery used to treat CPCs localized in the anterior part of the lateral ventricle is restricted to: (1) direct surgical removal (total or partial) of the cyst and/or (2) CT stereoendoscopic resection of the cyst wall using the bipolar coagulator and laser.[10] Stereotactic puncture is considered an inferior approach by some authors because it does not provide the opportunity to confirm the fenestration via direct visualization or permit the surgeon to perform multiple openings in the cyst.[25] Margetis and Souweidane regard an endoscopic approach to CPC treatment as the superior technique because there is no risk for shunt dependency and no potential operative morbidity

associated with craniotomy.[22] In 2000, Gangemi et al. conducted a small case series treating patients with intraventricular and paraventricular CSF cysts in which endoscopic fenestration demonstrated a success rate of more than 90%.[28] In that study, the authors took special considerations into account for their CPC cases depending on the size and location of the cyst. When the cyst was small or mid-sized and occupied only part of the ventricular cavity, it was approached through a homolateral occipital burr hole and treated via endoscopic fenestration from the homolateral enlarged ventricle to the cystic cavity; when the cyst was large and almost completely occupied the enlarged lateral ventricle, the authors found it easier to approach it through a contralateral, occipital burr hole and perform the fenestration from the contralateral, normal-sized ventricle.[28] This variation in technique was successful in treating the larger CPC cases the authors described in their paper: cyst size decreased and the foramen of Monro was successfully recanalized.[28] Very few subsequent case studies have been reported in the literature, but there have been several accounts of successful endoscopic cyst fenestration, cauterization, and removal that support Gangemi's findings and advocate the endoscopic approach as the primary treatment option for this pathology.[16,17,19,22,25]

Choroid plexus cysts appear to be more common in aneuploidy fetuses, especially those with trisomy 18.[14] In 44% to 50% of pregnancies with trisomy 18, antenatal ultrasonography reveals cysts of the choroid plexus.[29]

While there is a general consensus that cysts with diameter less than 5 mm may not be linked to aneuploidy, larger cysts in excess of 10 mm may indicate a higher risk and have clinical implications.[29] Some have proposed that every fetus with an isolated CPC undergo invasive genetic testing, but this stance is controversial due to the associated risk for pregnancy loss. In a study conducted by Gray et al. evaluating the prevalence of trisomy 18 in the setting of isolated fetal CPCs, the authors ultimately concluded that the discovery of CPCs in otherwise normal fetuses during the late second trimester did not, by itself, justify the risks of genetic amniocentesis.[30] The current guidelines for antenatal detection of a CPC include further testing for associated anomalies and genetic counseling.[16]

EPENDYMAL CYSTS

Ependymal cysts in adults were first described in a report written by Zehnder in 1938.[31,32] They are congenital, benign cysts that are typically found in the central white matter of the temporoparietal and frontal lobes.[3,31] Authors have reported finding these cysts most frequently in the supratentorial cerebral parenchyma, but they are also occasionally encountered in the juxtraventricular region, subarachnoid space, spinal subarachnoid space, and pons.[33] Ependymal cysts are very rare; as of 2011, there was no prevalence or incidence rate reported for this condition.[31] Excision is the preferable approach to treatment because puncturing the cyst wall or creating an opening into the lateral ventricle or subarachnoid space has been associated with cyst recurrence.[8,33]

Patients with ependymal cysts usually experience clinical symptoms that stem from neurological deficits related to the frontal or temporoparietal regions; they might also exhibit hemiparesis, seizures, increased intracranial pressure, chronic headache, or psychiatric manifestations.[3,33,34] Examples of psychiatric symptoms that have been associated with ependymal cyst cases include: confusion, memory deterioration, mental slowness, poor concentration, irritability, personality disturbances, and psychiatric manifestations.[33,35] In 1996, Pant et al. reported a case in which a patient with an ependymal cyst presented with psychiatric symptoms that could not be attributed to any definite pattern of psychiatric illness but had characteristics of both schizophrenia and depression.[33] It was a unique case because the patient presented with no other neurologic deficit, only a long history of psychosis that could not be alleviated with medication. After endoscopic resection of the ependymal cyst, the

patient's symptoms resolved almost completely. Several reports have indicated that ependymal cysts may also be involved in movement disorders, such as tremor, ballismus, hemiballismus, and choreoathetosis.[34,36] Symptoms generally present during adulthood and progress rapidly after onset.[33]

Ependymal cysts are characterized by a single layer of ciliated or nonciliated cuboidal or columnar epithelial cells directly abutting a gliotic neuropil or lying on a glial stroma.[34,37] The cells should demonstrate epithelial immunoreactivity for glial markers that are typical of ependymal epithelium, such as S-100 protein and GFAP.[23,34] Sharpe and Deck reported a case in which they observed a neuroepithelial cyst wall with a thin layer of astrocytic glial tissue that appeared to be lined with cells resembling both ependymal and choroid plexus epithelium.[38] These types of observations in conjunction with reports of neuroepithelial tumors demonstrating immunoreactivity to cytokeratins and GFAP have suggested to some authors that there might exist transitional cell types that have features of both the ependyma and the choroid plexus.[12] Cysts with an epithelial lining that rests directly on brain parenchyma or a layer of astroglia rather than a basement membrane and connective tissue are appropriately diagnosed as ependymal cysts.[3] According to Odake et al., the apparent absence of an ependymal lining should not exclude the diagnosis of an ependymal cyst because a severely stretched cyst wall could attenuate the lining in such a way that it might be difficult to identify without electromicroscopic confirmation.[11] CT analysis of ependymal cysts will likely reveal contents that are isodense with CSF and demonstrate the localized expansion of the trigone and lateral ventricle.[3,5,39] On CT there is usually little to no visualization of a cyst wall, but MRI should make it easier to detect.[3,39]

Ependymal cysts are hypothesized to be the end result of a developmental defect in which the ependyma is displaced into the cerebral substance or the subarachnoid space. Several mechanism have been proposed to explain exactly how this displacement occurs, including: (1) anomalous mantle layer formation that causes the ventricular diverticulum to pinch off and isolate an ependymal-lined pouch within the cerebral substance that eventually gives origin to the cysts and (2) the differentiation of spongioblastic cells into ependyma due to a primary encephaloclastic intracerebral defect occurring in early fetal life.[8,35,40-42] The mechanisms that potentially account for fluid accumulation within the cyst include:

active secretion, transcellular fluid transport (suggested by the presence of numerous pinocytotic vesicles), and passive transport drawing in water from the surrounding tissue due to cyst fluid hyperosmolality.[3,32,33,42]

REGARDING INTRAVENTRICULAR ARACHNOID CYSTS AND THEIR CLASSIFICATION

In 1979, Yeates and Enzmann presented the first report of an intraventricular arachnoid cyst.[43,44] They described a cyst with focal expansion of the lateral ventricle, attenuation values in the range of CSF, and a lack of communication with the ventricular system.[44] The authors postulated that the cyst originated from arachnoid tissue in the choroid plexus that had bulged into the lateral ventricle; ultimately, surgical findings confirmed that the cyst wall was composed of a gliotic outer layer and an arachnoid inner layer.[44] Since that time, other authors have presented similar cases over the years. In 1992, Martinez-Lage et al. described an outer connective membrane with gliotic elements of a reactive astrocytic nature and an inner layer lined by flattened cells of arachnoid origin with occasional arachnoid cell nests.[2] Nakase et al. also mentioned connective tissue and arachnoid cells in their contemporary report describing the wall of a lateral ventricle neuroepithelial cyst.[45] Pelletier et al. hypothesized that these sorts of intraventricular cysts are not technically of arachnoid origin because they appear to arise from the plexus; for that reason, the authors assert that it would be more accurate to describe these lesions as CPCs rather than arachnoid cysts.[26] Classifying arachnoid cysts as a type of neuroepithelial cyst is not wholly accurate for both pathophysiological and histological reasons. Unlike neuroepithelial cysts, arachnoid cysts that become symptomatic do so in early childhood; arachnoid cyst cells also test positive for epithelial membrane antigens and negative for neuroepithelial markers, such as GFAP, S-100 protein, and prealbumin.[3,46] MRI analysis of arachnoid cystic contents generally show a low protein pattern that is different from that of a colloid cyst, hemorrhagic cyst, and nonhemorrhagic tumoral cyst.[47] These factors markedly distinguish arachnoid cysts and seem to justify a distinction in their classification. There have been several attempts made to explain the presence of arachnoid cysts within the ventricles. Authors have suggested: (1) that the cysts are the result of the arachnoid membrane splitting, (2) the cysts form in response to the

agenesis of the temporal lobe, and (3) the cells originate from the ependymal layer of the tela choroidea covering the vascular mesenchyma, which later projects into the lateral ventricle through the choroid fissure as the choroid plexus.[2] In spite of all this useful speculation, a definitive answer has still not been reported.

CLINICAL CASES

Case 1

A 2-year-old male began complaining of headaches and developed right-sided mild weakness and poor coordination. A diagnostic brain MRI was done (Figs. 2 to 4) which demonstrated asymmetrical ventricles with left larger than right. Careful review demonstrated what appeared to be an atrial ventricular cyst causing mass effect. The decision to treat endoscopically was undertaken and he was taken to surgery. A left frontal approach was chosen (Fig. 5). At the time of surgery a ventriculostomy catheter was inserted and an opening pressure of 32 cm H_2O was obtained. A rigid endoscope was inserted into the cyst and a thick wall (Figs. 6 and 7) was noticed compressing the neural structures. The cyst was fenestrated using YAG laser and communication established with the ventricular system. Closing pressure was 3 cm H_2O (Figs. 8 to 15). The following day, an MRI showed decompression of the cyst and ventricles (Figs. 16 to 18) and such was the case at a 1-year follow-up MRI (Figs. 19A to D). The patient was asymptomatic and clinically stable.

Case 2

A 6-year-old female presented with severe headaches whenever she put her head forward and down. A diagnostic workup was negative for a specific lesion. However, headaches worsened with time and a decision to perform a spinal tap and a cisternogram was done. Her opening pressure was 15 cm H_2O but the cisternogram appeared to show an area that did not allow the intracisternal dye to enter near the right foramen of Monro. An endoscopic exploration was proposed and her parents agreed. At the time of surgery a large, sessile, mobile, and fluctuating CPC was encountered (Figs. 20 and 21). The cyst was easily cauterized (Fig. 22) and involuted using a YAG laser (Fig. 23). The patient became asymptomatic and has remained so for 10 years. Surgical length: 45 minutes; estimated blood loss: <5 cc; length of stay: 1 day.

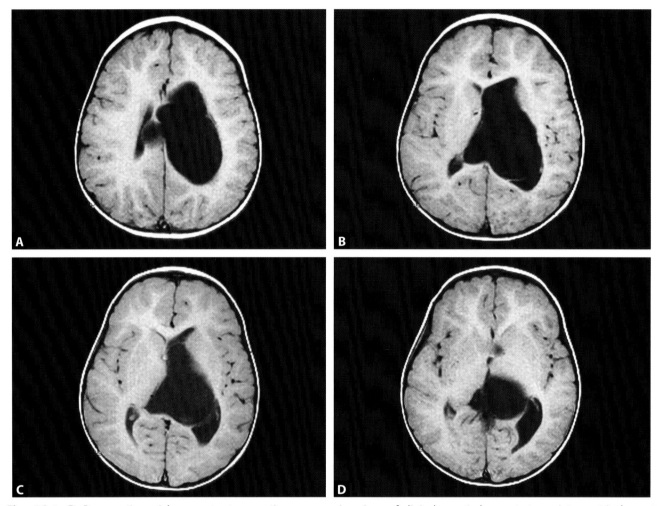

Figs. 2A to D: Preoperative axial noncontrast magnetic resonance imagings of clinical case 1 demonstrate an intraventricular cyst located on the left ventricle causing acute ventricular dilation and mass effect.

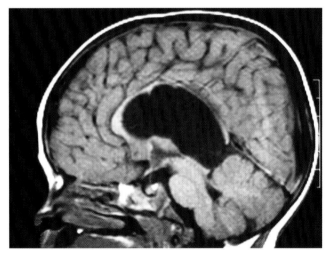

Fig. 3: Clinical case 1 preoperative sagittal magnetic resonance imaging shows marked ventricular dilation and corpus callosum stretching as well as compression.

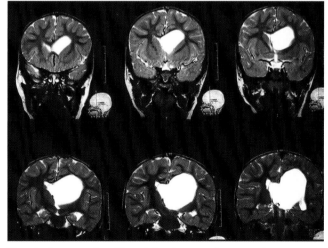

Fig. 4: Preoperative T2-weighted coronal magnetic resonance imaging shows significant left ventricular dilation secondary to large intraventricular cyst.

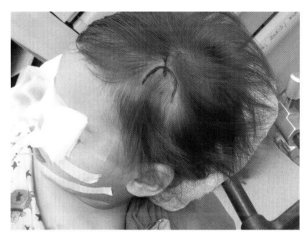

Fig. 5: Intraoperative setup showing a laterally placed left frontal approach.

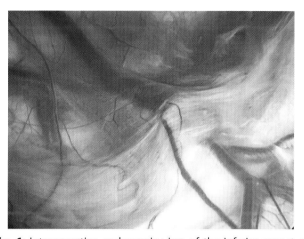

Fig. 6: Intraoperative endoscopic view of the inferior aspect of the cyst. A thick membrane is noticed enveloping venous and neural ventricular structures.

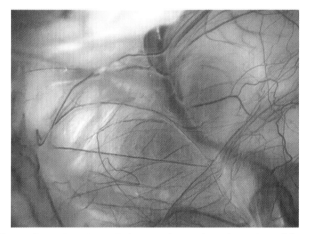

Fig. 7: Posterior view of the cyst located in the occipital horn causing mass effect on the ventricular wall, as seen on the magnetic resonance imaging scans.

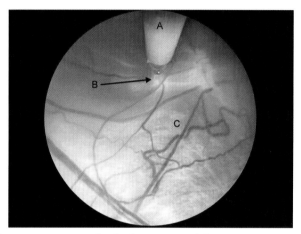

Fig. 8: In preparation for the fenestration of the cyst into the ventricular system, a YAG laser 500 micron fiber (A) is set and the localizing red beam (B) is seen on a vascularized area of the cyst wall (C).

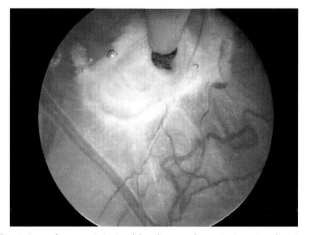

Fig. 9: In order to minimize bleeding and maximize visualization, the cyst wall is devascularized with the laser beam aimed at the wall vessels. At this point, no direct contact is made. Notice the blanching and disappearance of the vasculature.

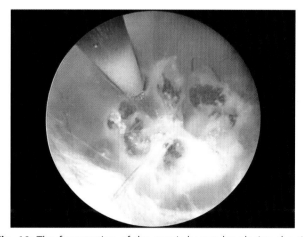

Fig. 10: The fenestration of the cyst is begun by placing the tip of the laser in direct contact with the cyst wall and delivering energy at about 10 watts. The maneuver is repeated sequentially and in clockwise fashion.

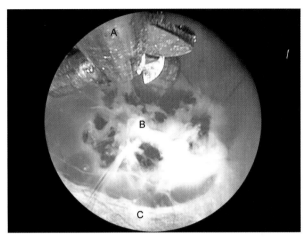

Fig. 11: Once the center has been devascularized and partially detached, a grasping or biopsy forceps (A) is used to remove the center (B) from the surrounding cyst wall (C).

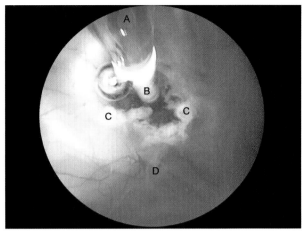

Fig. 12: Once a primary fenestration is performed, a Fogarty catheter (A) is inserted through the working channel of the endoscope and the deflated balloon (B) is placed inside the fenestrated wall (C) of the cyst wall (D).

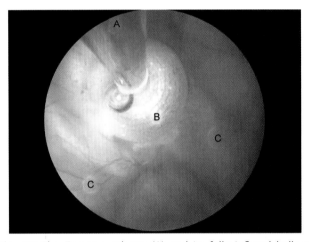

Fig. 13: The Fogarty catheter (A) and its fully inflated balloon (B) inside the fenestration. This maneuver allows for further expansion of the fenestration made on the cyst wall (C).

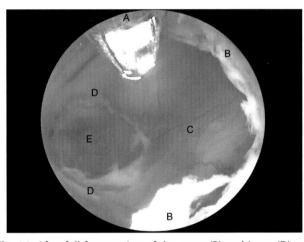

Fig. 14: After full fenestration of the outer (B) and inner (D) cyst walls, the two fenestrations (C and E) can be seen. The grasping forceps (A) is seen at the 12 o'clock position.

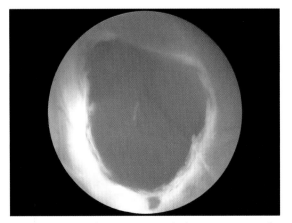

Fig. 15: Completed fenestration and decompression of intraventricular cyst.

Case 3

A 14-year-old female presented with chronic headaches and blurry vision. Physical examination was normal and negative for papilledema. A diagnostic MRI showed asymmetric, dilated ventricles and ventricular enlargement (Figs. 24 to 26). She was taken for surgery for a ventricular exploration and fenestration of a suspected intraventricular cyst. The ventricular system was approached using image guidance from the left superior parietal area (Fig. 27). A thick, vascularized membrane was encountered (Figs. 28 and 29). A YAG laser was used to create a fenestration into the cyst (Figs. 30 and 31) following cyst fenestration and

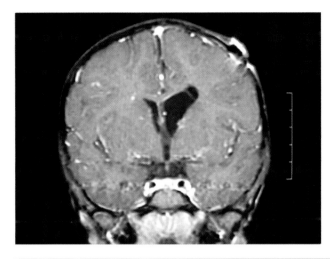

Fig. 16: After undergoing an intraventricular laser fenestration of the cyst a POD 1 coronal MRI shows entrance site on the left frontal area and decompression of the cyst at the level of foramen of Monro. (POD 1: Postoperative day 1; MRI: Magnetic resonance imaging).

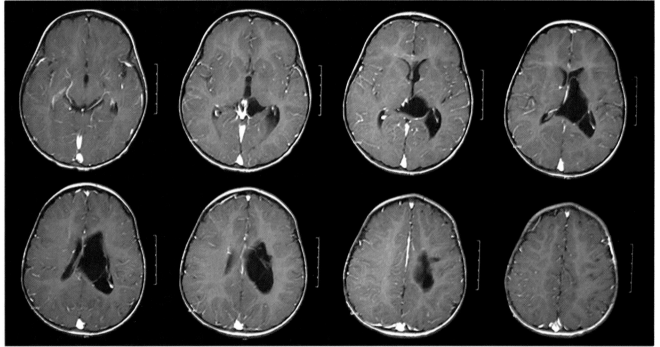

Fig. 17: Postoperative day 1 axial magnetic resonance imaging also shows decompression of cyst and fenestration into the occipital horn.

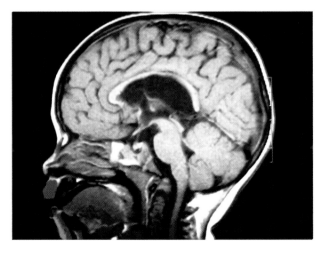

Fig. 18: Postoperative day 1 sagittal magnetic resonance imaging shows re-expansion of the body of the corpus callosum and less ventriculomegaly.

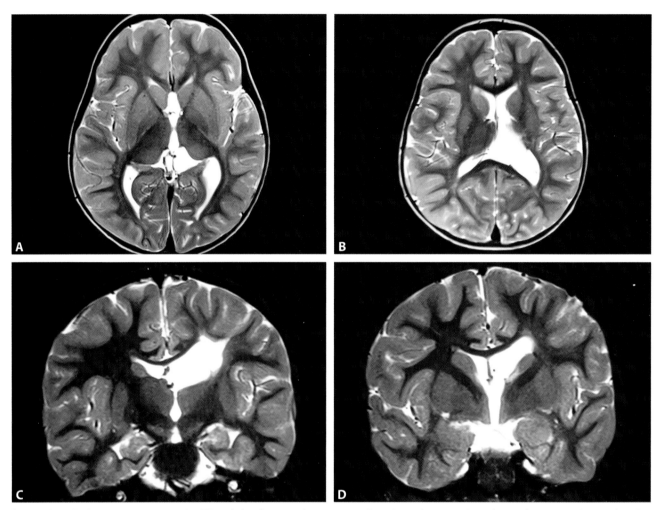

Figs. 19A to D: One-year postoperative T2-weighted magnetic resonance imagings show continued cyst decompression and patient remained asymptomatic.

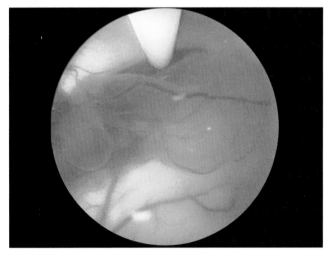

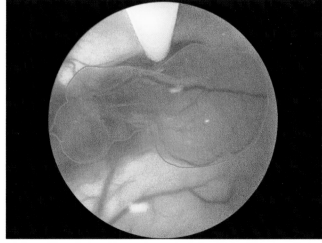

Fig. 20: Endoscopic view of patient, clinical case 2 who presented with a choroid plexus cyst near the right foramen of Monro. A diaphanous, vascularized membrane is difficult to fully visualize.

Fig. 21: The edges of the cyst have been traced in red, in order to improve visualization of its extension as it sits in front of the foramen of Monro.

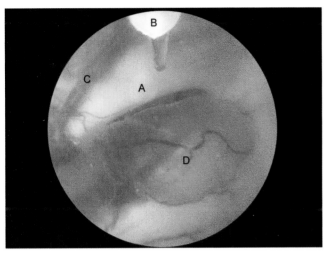

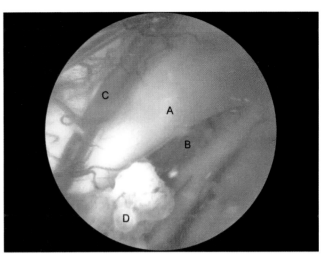

Fig. 22: The YAG laser fiber (B) is seen in the upper part of the image. The column of the right fornix (A) and a trace of the foramen of Monro are noted. The septal vein (C) and the choroid plexus cyst (D) are also seen.

Fig. 23: After full fulguration of the cyst (D) with the YAG laser, the cyst is seen shrunken and devascularized. The foramen of monro (B) is now open. The column of the fornix (A) and septal vein (C) are easily seen.

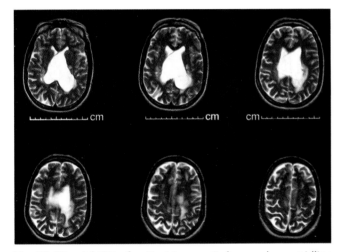

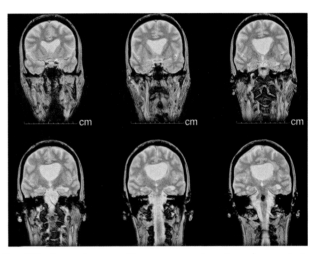

Fig. 24: T2 axial MRI of patient in case 3 shows a large midline intraventricular cyst.

Fig. 25: Coronal magnetic resonance imaging demonstrates marked enlargement of the ventricular system.

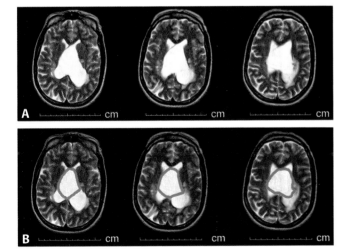

Figs. 26A and B: (A) Closer view of the ventricular systems shows the faint outline of an intraventricular cyst located posteriorly on the left ventricle. (B) The cyst has been outlined in red for improved visualization.

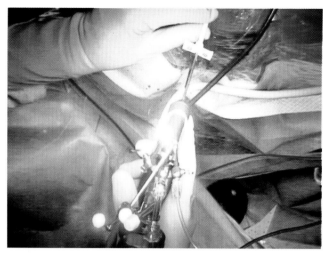

Fig. 27: The Oi endoscope has been adapted with image guidance tracker and is being inserted into the peel away introducer sheet via a frontal approach.

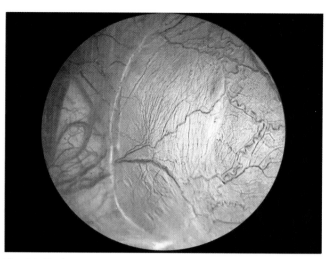

Fig. 28: Endoscopic view, upon entrance, of the cyst wall. Notice a thick and fibrous cyst wall which would be very difficult to puncture with a ventricular catheter.

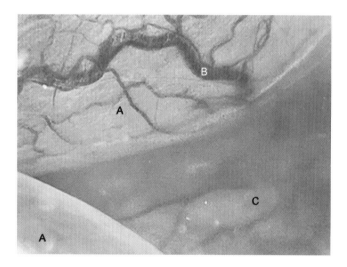

Fig. 29: Closer view shows the cyst wall (A) and cyst wall vessels (B). The ventricular system is seen in (C).

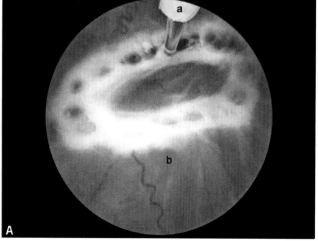

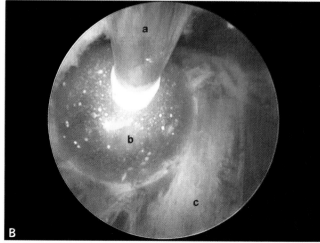

Figs. 30A and B: (A) The YAG laser (a) is being used in contracts mode to create serial and circumferential openings into the cyst wall (b) in order to create a larger fenestration. (B) Shows the fogarty catheter (a) with the balloon being fully inflated (b) in the fenestration of the cyst wall (c).

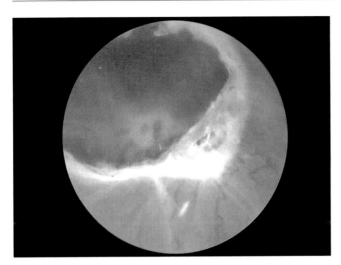

Fig. 31: The fenestration has been enlarged and allows full communication between the cyst interior and the ventricular system.

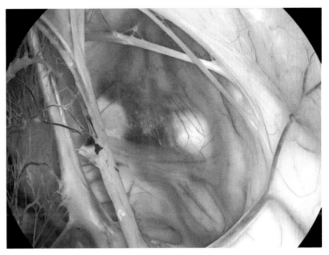

Fig. 32: The enlarged and distorted foramen of monro can be seen after the fenestration along with the contents of the anterior third ventricle.

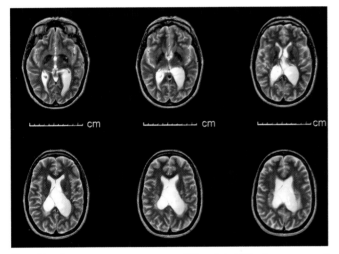

Fig. 33: One year post surgery T2 axial MRI shows a well decompressed ventricular system.

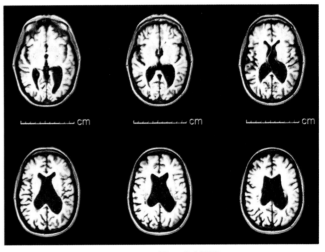

Fig. 34: One year post surgery T1 axial MRI.

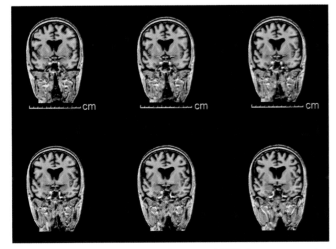

Fig. 35: One year post surgery T1 coronal MRI shows anatomical normalization.

decompression, the ventricular system, enlarged foramen of Monro, and third ventricle were easily visualized (Fig. 32). Postoperative MRIs showed decompression of cyst and normalization of ventricular size and shape (Figs. 33 to 35). The patient has remained asymptomatic 4 years later.

CONCLUSION

Although not particularly common, intraventricular cysts can become symptomatic and may require treatment. The advent of neuroendoscopic techniques has simplified their treatment. These cysts tend to have thick walls and are neither really amenable to shunting (difficulty getting the catheter into the cyst) nor to stereotactic drainage (difficulty puncturing cyst and maintaining drainage). Depending on the cyst type, they may be fulgurated (CPCs) or fenestrated. Our long-term results have been excellent with no mortalities or morbidities. Endoscopic management of these cysts is an excellent, safe, and effective treatment option.

REFERENCES

1. Osborn AG, Preece MT. Intracranial cysts: radiologic-pathologic correlation and imaging approach. Radiology. 2006;239(3):650-64.

2. Martinez-Lage JF, Poza M, Sola J, et al. Congenital arachnoid cyst of the lateral ventricles in children. Child's Nerv Syst. 1992;8(4):203-6.

3. Boockvar JA, Shafa R, Forman MS, et al. Symptomatic lateral ventricular ependymal cysts: criteria for distinguishing these rare cysts from other symptomatic cysts of the ventricles: case report. Neurosurgery. 2000;46(5):1229-32; discussion 1232-3.

4. Lach B, Scheithauer BW, Gregor A, et al. Colloid cyst of the third ventricle. A comparative immunohistochemical study of neuraxis cysts and choroid plexus epithelium. J Neurosurg. 1993;78(1):101-11.

5. New PF, Davis KR. Intraventricular noncolloid neuroepithelial cysts. AJNR Am J Neuroradiol. 1981;2(6):569-76.

6. Ciricillo SF, Davis RL, Wilson CB. Neuroepithelial cysts of the posterior fossa. Case report. J Neurosurg. 1990;72(2):302-5.

7. Shuangshoti S, Netsky MG. Histogenesis of choroid plexus in man. Am J Anatomy. 1966;118(1):283-316.

8. MacGregor BJ, Gawler J, South JR. Intracranial epithelial cysts. Report of two cases. J Neurosurg. 1976;44(1):109-15.

9. Shuangshoti S. Calcified congenital arachnoid cyst with heterotopic neuroglia in wall. J Neurol Neurosurg Psychiat. 1978;41(1):88-94.

10. Pařízek J, Jakubec J, Hobza V, et al. Choroid plexus cyst of the left lateral ventricle with intermittent blockage of the foramen of Monro, and initial invagination into the III ventricle in a child. Child's Nerv Syst. 1998;14(12):700-8.

11. Odake G, Tenjin H, Murakami N. Cyst of the choroid plexus in the lateral ventricle: case report and review of the literature. Neurosurgery. 1990;27(3):470-6.

12. Mannoji H, Becker LE. Ependymal and choroid plexus tumors. Cytokeratin and GFAP expression. Cancer. 1988;61(7):1377-85.

13. Kouno M, Kumanishi T, Washiyama K, et al. An immunohistochemical study of cytokeratin and glial fibrillary acidic protein in choroid plexus papilloma. Acta Neuropathol. 1988;75(3):317-20.

14. Kennedy KA, Carey JC. Choroid plexus cysts: significance and current management practices. Seminars in ultrasound, CT, and MR. 1993;14(1):23-30.

15. Chudleigh P, Pearce JM, Campbell S. The prenatal diagnosis of transient cysts of the fetal choroid plexus. Prenat Diagn. 1984;4(2):135-7.

16. Filardi TZ, Finn L, Gabikian P, et al. Treatment of intermittent obstructive hydrocephalus secondary to a choroid plexus cyst. J Neurosurg Pediatrics. 2009;4(6):571-4.

17. Chamczuk AJ, Grand W. Endoscopic cauterization of a symptomatic choroid plexus cyst at the foramen of Monro: case report. Neurosurgery. 2010;66(6 Suppl Operative):376-7.

18. Hatashita S, Takagi S, Sakakibara T. Choroid plexus cyst of the lateral ventricle in an elderly man. Case report. J Neurosurg. 1984;60(2):435-7.

19. Azab WA, Mijalcic RM, Aboalhasan AA, et al. Endoscopic management of a choroid plexus cyst of the third ventricle: case report and documentation of dynamic behavior. Child's Nerv Syst. 2015;31(5):815-9.

20. Giorgi C. Symptomatic cyst of the choroid plexus of the lateral ventricle. Neurosurgery. 1979;5(1 Pt 1):53-6.

21. Dempsey RJ, Chandler WF. Choroid plexus cyst in the lateral ventricle causing obstructive symptoms in an adult. Surg Neurol. 1981;15(2):116-9.

22. Margetis K, Souweidane MM. Endoscopic treatment of intraventricular cystic tumors. World Neurosurg. 2013;79(2 Suppl):S19.e1-e11.

23. Coca S, Martinez A, Vaquero J, et al. Immunohistochemical study of intracranial cysts. Histol Histopathol. 1993;8(4):651-4.

24. Matsushima T, Inoue T, Takeshita I, et al. Choroid plexus papillomas: an immunohistochemical study with particular reference to the coexpression of prealbumin. Neurosurgery. 1988;23(3):384-9.

25. Nahed BV, Darbar A, Doiron R, et al. Acute hydrocephalus secondary to obstruction of the foramen of monro and cerebral aqueduct caused by a choroid plexus cyst in the lateral ventricle. Case report. J Neurosurg. 2007;107(3 Suppl):236-9.

26. Pelletier J, Milandre L, Peragut JC, et al. Intraventricular choroid plexus "arachnoid" cyst. MRI findings. Neuroradiology. 1990;32(6):523-5.

27. Hanbali F, Fuller GN, Leeds NE, et al. Choroid plexus cyst and chordoid glioma. Report of two cases. Neurosurg Focus. 2001;10(6):E5.

28. Gangemi M, Maiuri F, Godano U, et al. Endoscopic treatment of para- and intraventricular cerebrospinal fluid cysts. Minim Invas Neurosurg. 2000;43(3):153-8.

29. Sasani M, Afsharian R, Sasani H, et al. A large choroid plexus cyst diagnosed with magnetic resonance imaging in utero: a case report. Cases J. 2009;2:7098.

30. Gray DL, Winborn RC, Suessen TL, et al. Is genetic amniocentesis warranted when isolated choroid plexus cysts are found? Prenat Diagn. 1996;16(11):983-90.

31. Saini AG, Singhi P, Bharti B, et al. Ependymal brain cyst with posterior cerebral artery infarct. Indian J Pediat. 2013;80(6):509-12.

32. Friede RL, Yasargil MG. Supratentorial intracerebral epithelial (ependymal) cysts: review, case reports, and fine structure. J Neurol Neurosurg Psychiatr. 1977;40(2):127-37.

33. Pant B, Uozumi T, Hirohata T, et al. Endoscopic resection of intraventricular ependymal cyst presenting with psychosis. Surg Neurol. 1996;46(6):573-6; discussion 576-8.

34. Colnat-Coulbois S, Marchal JC. Thalamic ependymal cyst presenting with tremor. Child's Nerv Syst. 2005;21(10):933-5.

35. Bouch DC, Mitchell I, Maloney AF. Ependymal lined paraventricular cerebral cysts; a report of three cases. J Neurol Neurosurg Psychiatr. 1973;36(4):611-7.

36. Bejar JM, Kepes J, Koller WC. Hemiballism and tremor due to ependymal cyst. Mov Disord 1992;7(4):370-2.

37. Andrews BT, Halks-Miller M, Berger MS, et al. Neuroepithelial cysts of the posterior fossa: pathogenesis and report of two cases. Neurosurgery. 1984;15(1):91-5.

38. Sharpe JA, Deck JH. Neuroepithelial cyst of the fourth ventricle. Case report. J Neurosurg. 1977;46(6):820-4.

39. Czervionke LF, Daniels DL, Meyer GA, et al. Neuroepithelial cysts of the lateral ventricles: MR appearance. AJNR Am J Neuroradiol. 1987;8(4):609-13.

40. Rand BO, Foltz EL, Alvord EC Jr. Intracranial Telencephalic Meningo-encephalocele containing choroid plexus. J Neuropathol Exp Neurol. 1964;23:293-305.

41. Patrick BS. Ependymal cyst of the sylvian fissure: case report. J Neurosurg. 1971;35(6):751-4.

42. Jakubiak P, Dunsmore RH, Beckett RS. Supratentorial brain cysts. J Neurosurg. 1968;28(2):129-36.

43. Nakase H, Hisanaga M, Hashimoto S, et al. Intraventricular arachnoid cyst: report of two cases. J Neurosurg. 1988; 68(3):482-6.

44. Yeates A, Enzmann D. An intraventricular arachnoid cyst. J Comput Assist Tomogr. 1979;3(5):697-700.

45. Nakase H, Ishida Y, Tada T, et al. Neuroepithelial cyst of the lateral ventricle. Clinical features and treatment. Surg Neurol. 1992;37(2):94-100.

46. Inoue T, Matsushima T, Fukui M, et al. Immunohistochemical study of intracranial cysts. Neurosurgery. 1988; 23(5):576-81.

47. Kurokawa Y, Sohma T, Tsuchita H, et al. A case of intraventricular arachnoid cyst. How should it be treated? Child's Nerv Syst. 1990;6(6):365-7.

CHAPTER 16

Risks and Complications

David N Garza, David F Jimenez

INTRODUCTION

There are a wide range of possible complications associated with endoscopic neurosurgery. These include: arrhythmia, hypertension, increased cranial pressure, ventriculitis, cerebrospinal fluid (CSF) leakage, wound infection, hygroma/hematoma, venous/arterial hemorrhage, respiratory dysfunction, delayed emergence, Parinaud syndrome, hemianopia, hemiparesis, nerve palsy, diabetes insipidus (DI), syndrome of inappropriate antidiuretic hormone secretion (SIADH), and the disturbance of temperature regulation or electrolyte regulation.[1,2] Infection is a relatively infrequent complication; its incidence ranges from 0% to 5%.[3] The overall rate of neural injury is higher, ranging between 3% and 4%.[4] Because maintaining hemostasis using endoscopic instrumentation can be difficult, hemorrhage is considered the most worrisome complication of all.[5] Intraventricular bleeding from small subependymal vessels due to traumatic injury caused by endoscopic instrumentation impact is the most frequently reported hemorrhagic complication.[5] Most neuroendoscopic complications are transient; they might resolve spontaneously or through medical intervention. The complications that present after a month tend to persist and remain for 6 months or longer.[2] The overall complication rate for all neuroendoscopic procedures is somewhat difficult to pinpoint because there are so many types of surgery to consider and so few large case series that include a significant number of procedures beyond endoscopic third ventriculostomy (ETV). Variation in classification and methodological organization within the literature can also makes it difficult to compare the results of different studies. For this reason, it is advisable for future authors to be

as precise and explicit as possible when describing their criteria for complication categorization and their definition of any reported rates. The goal of this chapter is to review the literature and make the reader aware of these possible problems in their practice.

GENERAL CONCEPTS

In their 1995 review of 173 neuroendoscopic procedures, Teo et al. reported an overall complication rate of 19%. Of the events studied, 13% were considered clinically "insignificant" complications and 7% were considered "significant".[6] These events were deemed insignificant if they incurred no overtly negative clinical sequelae. Intraoperative hemorrhage that could be managed without the need for transfusion or resultant neurological deficit was also considered insignificant.[6] In a 2004 study examining 485 neuroendoscopic procedures, Beems and Grotenhuis reported an overall complication rate of 9.3% and a mortality rate of 0.2%.[2] The authors further distinguished complications based on whether they were short term (resolving before the first postsurgical month) or long term (persisting after the first postsurgical month). Out of the total number of complications recorded, 36 (7.4%) were transient and only nine (1.6%) were permanent.[2] It should be noted that the authors did not analyze intraoperative complications because they believed they were beyond the scope of their report.[2] The authors suggested that the most critical complications they documented during the course of their study were not the direct result of the endoscopic procedure. They believe that it is more accurate to attribute these complications to the danger of vascular damage and intractable bleeding endemic to the ventricular approach itself.[2] Whether they are regarded as lethal, transient, or "clinically insignificant," all complications should be taken into careful consideration because of their potential to affect recovery time and overall patient well-being.

Teo et al. observed that while clinically insignificant complications appeared to diminish with additional surgical experience, clinically significant complications seemed to occur regardless of surgical training level.[6] However, a study conducted by Schroeder et al. suggested that surgical experience did help reduce the rate of permanent and lethal complications. When comparing the complications for their entire series (344 procedures) with the complications of the last 100 procedures performed, the authors found a decrease in mortality and permanent morbidity from 0.9% and 1.3% to 0% and 0%, respectively.[7] Aside from intensive surgical training, careful patient selection, preoperative imaging studies, intraoperative systemic hemodynamic monitoring, and clear communication with the anesthesiologist can also help prevent complications from occurring.[1,5]

With regard to patient selection, the ideal candidate for surgery would have large ventricles, a third ventricle wider than the diameter of the scope/sheath, an attenuated third ventricular floor, a capacious interpeduncular cistern, and no aberrant anatomy.[8] Some authors have specifically recommended a minimum third ventricular width of 7–10 mm.[9] Surgical planning can help mitigate some of the difficulty engendered by narrow ventricles. Under such circumstances, a better approach might involve a more medially placed burr hole with a slightly more vertical trajectory.[9] A history of post-infectious or post-hemorrhagic hydrocephalus are generally considered contraindications for surgeons who do not have sufficient experience with the neuroendoscopic tools and techniques.[9] However, some authors contend that endoscopic surgery can be safely performed in small ventricles if sufficient precautions are taken. It is the senior author's practice to use image guidance when operating in small ventricles to minimize the possibility of complications. A clear surgical field of view is mandatory for a successful procedure and outcome. The use of constant irrigation is necessary to keep a clear field of view. Care must be taken by the surgeon to assure that whatever amount of irrigant fluid is being introduced in the brain, that the same amount exits the brain contemporaneously. Failure to do so can lead to catastrophic consequences. If fluid does not leave at the same rate, it will accumulate and compress the brain and ultimately lead to brain herniation. If the

anesthesiologist alerts the surgeon of an acute Cushing's triad event (hypertension, bradycardia, and irregular respirations), attention should immediately to the outflow cannula and assuring that irrigant fluid is adequately exiting the ventricles. If none is seen, the cannula should be quickly repositioned until fluid is expressed.

ENDOSCOPIC THIRD VENTRICULOSTOMY

Exposure to neurologic complications during ETV is higher than the risk of a single-shunt operation, but that higher risk is offset by the opportunity for the patient to achieve shunt independence and avoid the cumulative morbidity that shunt failure inevitably entails.[9] The overall complication rate for ETV, the most frequently performed intraventricular endoscopic procedure, varies widely in the literature. Reported rates have ranged from 0% to 20%, but some authors suspect that incidences of severe surgical complication often go unreported, especially those involving serious vascular injury.[3,5,10-13] Possible complications associated with ETV include: bradycardia, asystole, visual obscuration, damage to the fornices, damage to the hypothalamus, vascular damage, subdural hygroma, cranial neuropathies, seizures, infection, intracerebral hemorrhage, postoperative neurological deficit, and subdural hematoma.[8] CSF leak is a rarely reported complication in the literature, but close observation is highly recommended because it is frequently signifies ETV failure.[9]

Damage to the hypothalamus is the most commonly reported ETV complication; it is associated with a series of other complications, including: permanent or transient DI, amenorrhea, loss of thirst, death, hyperphagia, drowsiness, hyperkalemia, hyponatremia, and a decrease in insulin-like growth factor.[8] Direct mechanical effect on the hypothalamus has also been linked to the bradycardia and asystole sometimes observed when surgeons perforate the third ventricular floor or enlarge the ventriculostomy; however, a dramatic increase in ventricular pressure caused by trapped irrigation fluid could also elicit those intraoperative complications.[9] By limiting the irrigation rate and ensuring one port of the endoscope is open for fluid egress, surgeons can decrease the risk of hemodynamic instability.[9]

The use of normal saline solution for irrigation also plays a role in hypothalamic dysfunction.[9] Because saline lacks the appropriate pH, osmolality, and concentration of inorganic salts that are conducive to healthy neural tissue function, prolonged exposure to this solution in a closed environment can bring about a wide range of deleterious effects, including brain damage.[14] Lactated Ringer's solution and artificial CSF fluid are considered superior neurosurgical irrigants, especially during endoscopic procedures or protracted operations that require significantly more irrigation.[14]

The context of an ETV certainly plays a role in the sort of complications a surgeon might expect to encounter during surgery. In their study examining the complication rates of several neuroendoscopic procedures, Beems and Grotenhuis split ETV procedures into two categories: one with biopsy and one without biopsy. Patients who underwent ETV in combination with endoscopic biopsy had more complications while other procedures hardly demonstrated any permanent complications. The authors ultimately concluded that biopsy procedures that accompanied endoscopic treatment were the elements primarily responsible for increasing the number of complications among ETV patients.[2]

The most dangerous and life-threatening complication associated with ETV is arterial hemorrhage from the basilar artery or its perforators.[7,8] MRI studies have demonstrated that the location of the basil artery bifurcation is variable; it can be in anterior to the mammillary bodies, juxtaposed to the dorsum sella, or somewhere in between those locations.[8] Because of this variability, surgeon are advised to inspect preoperative CT scans or sagittal MR images in order to realize the individual relation of the basilar artery to the floor of the third ventricle in order to better avoid vascular and neural damage.[7] If there is a thinning area of the third ventricular floor that permits visualization of the basilar artery complex, the procedure can be safely performed.[9] If the floor is opaque, the risk of injury increases, particularly in the hands of inexperienced surgeons. Under those circumstances, a microvascular Doppler probe could be employed to help localize the basilar artery.[15,16]

CYSTS, TUMOR BIOPSY, AND MICROVASCULAR DECOMPRESSION

In their 2006 report, Nowoslawska et al. indicated that neuroendoscopic techniques were most suited to the treatment of arachnoid cysts when the connection between the lumen of the cyst and the CSF cisterns was of good quality.[17] The complications observed among their 44 patients treated with neuroendoscopic techniques included five children with CSF liquorrhea from postoperative wounds (11%), two children with irritation of the third nerve caused by the Fogarty catheter (4.5%), two children with subdural hematoma (4.5%), one child with central nervous system infection (2.3%), and one child who experienced intensive intraoperative bleeding (2.3%).[17] A slightly larger study focused on the treatment of arachnoid cysts was conducted by Oertel et al. in 2006. The authors found an overall postoperative complication rate of 16% and only one case of permanent deficit (2%).[18] They had to abandon four cases (7%) because they were unable to identify anatomic landmarks using endoscopic tools.[18] Venous hemorrhage was the only reported intraoperative complication. Reported postoperative complications included: seizure, transient trochlear nerve palsy, transient oculomotor nerve palsy, CSF fistula, epidural hematoma, subdural hygroma, subdural hematoma, transient DI, permanent DI, and meningitis. Hemorrhage is especially precarious because it can easily obscure the surgeon's view during surgery. To mitigate this complication, it is important for the surgeon to coagulate the fragile arachnoidal blood vessels in the entry zone to prevent bleeding caused by operating sheath movement.[7]

In their 2014 retrospective analysis reviewing the neuroendoscopic approach to colloid cyst resection, Sribnick et al. reported a complication rate of about 21%.[19] Among their 56 patients, the authors observed the following postoperative complications: transient short-term memory loss (11%), sustained memory loss (11%), infection (5.4%), transient hyponatremia (3.6%), deep vein thrombosis (1.8%), and hematoma (1.8%).[19] There were three deaths, but only two could be attributed to cyst removal (3.6%).[19] Several of these rates were comparable to previous findings in the literature. In 2006, Horn et al. reported an overall complication rate of 25% and a neurological complication rate of 11%.[20] Their reported rate of infection was 0%. In their 2007 paper, Grondin et al. reported only one complication out of 25 procedures (4%); a patient suffered an injury to the internal capsule with subsequent hemiparesis and a pulmonary embolism.[21] For colloid cysts, the risk of severe venous hemorrhage is high when the cyst is firmly adhered to the roof of the third ventricle and total capsule removal is attempted.[7]

Grondin et al. included a systematic review of endoscopic colloid cyst resection from 1994 to 2005 in their paper. After looking at data for 157 patients from studies ranging in size from one to 25 participants, they found only 13 patients with complications (8.3%), five of which were deemed major (3.2%) and eight minor (5.1%).[21]

Major complications included: hemiparesis, pulmonary embolus, bacterial meningitis, ventriculitis, bone flap infection, intracerebral hemorrhage, intraventricular hemorrhage, chronic seizure disorder, permanent neurological deficit, and death. Minor complications included: CSF leak, wound infection, aseptic meningitis, stitch granuloma, isolated seizure, subdural effusion, and transient neurological deficit (except hemiparesis).

In their paper discussing the management of symptomatic septum pellucidum cysts, Meng et al. reported that their team experienced fewer complications during endoscopic pellucidotomy compared to other types of endoscopic surgery. There was only one instance of bleeding in their ten patient series, which the authors attributed to their initial lack of experience.[22] Cai et al. reported similar findings endorsing the endoscopic approach to surgery. In their 12 patient series describing neuroendoscopic fenestration as a treatment for monoventricular hydrocephalus, the authors observed no severe complications.[23]

In their retrospective analysis of seven centers performing neuroendoscopic biopsies over a span of 10 years, Oppido et al. reported several minor complications that did not affect more than one or two patients each: epilepsy, hydrocephalus, meningitis, transient Parinaud syndrome, and intracerebral hematoma subsequent to ventricular puncture.[24] The only major complications they observed were eight cases of ventricular hemorrhage (13%). A study conducted by Giannetti et al. expressed similar findings. Among 50 patients who underwent endoscopic biopsy procedures, there were three hemorrhages (6%), two infections (4%), and one death (2%).[25] In both these studies, hemorrhage was the most common complication. Needle biopsies carry an inherent risk for bleeding; however, those incidents can usually be managed using bipolar cautery and continuous irrigation with lactated Ringer's solution.[2] Surgeons should also ensure that an outflow channel is open in order to avoid a dangerous increase intracranial pressure (ICP).[7]

The endoscopic approach to MVD for trigeminal neuralgia (TGN) has demonstrated an excellent record of patient safety. A study conducted by Chen et al. in 2008 evaluated 167 patients treated using the endoscopic approach to surgery. They reported four cases of cerebral hemorrhage (2.40%) and five CSF fluid leaks (2.99%); there were no deaths and no infection.[26] Similar findings have been reported by other authors. Kabil et al. compared the endoscopic and microscopic approaches to surgery in their 2005 study and found no serious complications or mortality.[27] In their study evaluating 20 patients who underwent endoscopic vascular decompression for TGN, hemifacial spasm (HFS), and cochleovestibular nerve compression syndrome (CNCS), Artz et al. observed no major complications. Within the TGN group, no patient experienced postoperative hearing loss, dizziness, facial weakness, or CSF leak; there was one instance of wound dehiscence.[28]

CONCLUSION

Like many other neurosurgical procedures, endoscopic surgery provides the patient with a great option at treating their problems. However, because of the delicate nature of these procedures, appropriate precautions should be undertaken. If care is taken to plan and execute these procedures, endoscopy can yield excellent results and superior outcomes to conventional treatment methods.

REFERENCES

1. Deutsch N. Challenges during pediatric endoscopic neurosurgery. In: Brambrink AM, Kirsch JR (Eds). Essentials of Neurosurgical Anesthesia and Critical Care. Berlin: Springer; 2012. pp. 539-45.
2. Beems T, Grotenhuis JA. Long-term complications and definition of failure of neuroendoscopic procedures. Child's Nerv Syst. 2004;20:868-77.
3. Chesler DA, Jallo GI. Iatrogenic and infectious complications. In: Rocco CD, Turgut M, Jallo G, Martinez-Lage JF (Eds). Complications of CSF Shunting in Hydrocephalus. Berlin: Springer; 2015. pp. 269-75.
4. Rehder R, Cohen AR. Complications of endoscopic third ventriculostomy. In: Rocco CD, Pang D, Rutka JT (Eds). Textbook of Pediatric Neurosurgery. Berlin: Springer; 2017. pp. 1-22.
5. Cinalli G, Spennato P, Ruggiero C, et al. Complications following endoscopic intracranial procedures in children. Child's Nerv Syst. 2007;23:633-44.
6. Teo C, Rahman S, Boop FA, et al. Complications of endoscopic neurosurgery. Child's Nerv Syst. 1996;12:248-53.
7. Schroeder HW, Oertel J, Gaab MR. Incidence of complications in neuroendoscopic surgery. Child's Nerv Syst. 2004;20:878-83.
8. Teo C. Complications of endoscopic third ventriculostomy. In: Cinalli G, Sainte-Rose C, Maixner WJ (Eds). Pediatric Hydrocephalus. Berlin: Springer; 2005. pp. 411-20.
9. Walker M. Complications of third ventriculostomy. Neurosurg Clin North Am. 2004;15:61-6.
10. Schroeder HW, Niendorf WR, Gaab MR. Complications of endoscopic third ventriculostomy. J Neurosurg. 2002; 96:1032-40.

11. Drake JM. The surgical management of pediatric hydrocephalus. Neurosurgery. 2008;62:SHC633-42.

12. Buxton N, Punt J. Cerebral infarction after neuroendoscopic third ventriculostomy: case report. Neurosurgery. 2000;46:999-1001.

13. Abtin K, Thompson BG, Walker ML. Basilar Artery Perforation as a Complication of Endoscopic Third Ventriculostomy. Pediatr Neurosurg. 1998;28:35-41.

14. Kazim SF, Enam SA, Shamim MS. Possible detrimental effects of neurosurgical irrigation fluids on neural tissue: An evidence based analysis of various irrigants used in contemporary neurosurgical practice. Int J Surg. 2010;8: 586-90.

15. Cartmill M, Vloeberghs M. The use of transendoscopic Doppler ultrasound as a safety-enhancing measure during neuroendoscopic third ventriculostomy. Eur J Pediatr Surg. 1999;9:50-1.

16. Schmidt RH. Use of microvascular Doppler probe to avoid basilar artery injury during endoscopic third ventriculostomy. J Neurosurg. 1999;90:156-9.

17. Nowosławska E, Polis L, Kaniewska D, et al. Neuroendoscopic techniques in the treatment of arachnoid cysts in children and comparison with other operative methods. Child's Nerv Syst. 2006;22:599-604.

18. Oertel JM, Baldauf J, Schroeder HW, et al. Endoscopic cystoventriculostomy for treatment of paraxial arachnoid cysts. J Neurosurg. 2009;110:792-9.

19. Sribnick EA, Dadashev VY, Miller BA, et al. Neuroendoscopic colloid cyst resection: a case cohort with follow-up and patient satisfaction. World Neurosurg. 2014;81:584-93.

20. Horn EM, Feiz-Erfan I, Bristol RE, et al. Treatment options for third ventricular colloid cysts: comparison of open microsurgical versus endoscopic resection. Neurosurgery. 2007;60:613-8; discussion 618-20.

21. Grondin RT, Hader W, MacRae ME, et al. Endoscopic versus microsurgical resection of third ventricle colloid cysts. Can J Neurol Sci. 2007;34:197-207.

22. Meng H, Feng H, Le F, et al. Neuroendoscopic management of symptomatic septum pellucidum cysts. Neurosurgery. 2006;59:278-83; discussion 278-83.

23. Cai Q, Song P, Chen Q, et al. Neuroendoscopic fenestration of the septum pellucidum for monoventricular hydrocephalus. Clin Neurol Neurosurg. 2013;115:976-80.

24. Oppido PA, Fiorindi A, Benvenuti L, et al. Neuroendoscopic biopsy of ventricular tumors: a multicentric experience. Neurosurgical Focus. 2011;30:E2.

25. Giannetti AV, Alvarenga AY, de Lima TO, et al. Neuroendoscopic biopsy of brain lesions: accuracy and complications. J Neurosurg. 2015;122:34-9.

26. Chen MJ, Zhang WJ, Yang C, et al. Endoscopic neurovascular perspective in microvascular decompression of trigeminal neuralgia. J Craniomaxillofac Surg. 2008;36:456-61.

27. Kabil M, Eby J, Shahinian H. Endoscopic vascular decompression versus microvascular decompression of the trigeminal nerve. Minim Invasive Neurosurg. 2005;48: 207-12.

28. Artz GJ, Hux FJ, LaRouere MJ, et al. Endoscopic vascular decompression. Otol Neurotol. 2008;29:995-1000.

Index

Page numbers followed by *f* refer to figure.